TOTAL REJUVENATION

From Skincare to Scalpel

Barry J. Cohen, MD, FACS

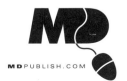

MDPUBLISH.COM

ISBN: 0-9748997-0-4

Printed in the United States of America.

Designed by Andrew Patapis

Illustrations by Jil Gordon

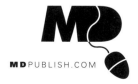

MD PUBLISH.COM   350 Fifth Avenue, Suite 7619 | New York, New York 10118

About the Author

Barry J. Cohen, MD, FACS is a Board Certified Plastic Surgeon, a Diplomate of the American Board of Plastic Surgery, and a Fellow of the American College of Surgeons. He practices all aspects of aesthetic plastic and reconstructive surgery, with a special interest in innovative cosmetic procedures of the face, body and breasts. His private practice is located in the Washington, D.C. area. Dr. Cohen graduated from the prestigious Cornell University with a Bachelor of Arts in Biochemistry. He went on to complete his medical school training at Georgetown University. He then served as a general surgery resident at the renowned trauma center at the Washington Hospital Center, where he received numerous awards for both his clinical and research skills. He completed his training in New York at The Long Island Plastic Surgical Group. That group, founded in the 1950s, is the largest plastic surgery group in the United States. In addition to his broad clinical training, Dr. Cohen has published numerous articles in the field of plastic surgery. Dr. Cohen is the founder and senior partner of the Washington Plastic Surgery Group, which has four plastic and reconstructive surgeons in four offices located in Chevy Chase, Rockville, and Annapolis, Maryland, and McLean, Virginia. The Washington Plastic Surgery Group provided the impetus for a medispa, where cosmetic surgery, skincare, and state-of-the-art face and body treatments will be merged into one comprehensive facility offering the most advanced menu of services to both women and men.

In 1978, Dr. Cohen founded Innovative Programming Associates (IPA), a software firm which began by designing custom software applications. Under Dr. Cohen's direction, the company has evolved into a world leader in the complete automation of the preclinical testing of drugs. IPA's software is used by numerous Fortune 500 pharmaceutical companies and government agencies, as well as private firms throughout the world.

As founder and chief executive officer of TotalSkinCare.com since 1998, Dr. Cohen has made available via the Internet medically formulated, nonprescription, skin care products that were previously available only through plastic surgeons' and dermatologists' offices. TotalSkinCare.com offers the most respected names in physician-grade skin care products.

Dr. Cohen was named as a Top Doctor in *The Washingtonian* and *Washington Consumers Checkbook*. He hosted a popular radio program in the Washington, D.C. area for several years, and is frequently the subject of media profiles.

To my Father,
who while alive, taught me about joie de vivre, *and*
by example, the importance of respecting my elders;

To my Mother,
who taught me the value of a strong work ethic and
by example, the importance of charity, humility,
and generosity;

To my wife Liza,
who has added untold spice to my life while serving
as my sounding board, cheerleader, and mother to
four incredibly wonderful and beautiful children;

To my children, Jason, Jordan, Erica, and Courtney,
who have added life to my years;

To my siblings Mort and Elaine,
who love me unconditionally;

And to G-d,
whom I acknowledge daily as the source of all of my
wealth, honor, and fortune.

Acknowledgements

To my talented partners, Adam Tattelbaum, Bennett Yang, and Frederick Watkins, whom I am lucky to call friends as well as associates. Thanks for always being there and supporting me on the wild ride we call the Washington Plastic Surgery Group. To my staff, especially Dica Cipu, who is always there and without whom I could not accomplish half the things I do. To Don Smith, Dr. Keith Moffat, Dr. William Fouty, Dr. Marion Jordan, Dr. Max Cohen, Dr. Roger Simpson, and Dr. Vincent DiGregorio — thanks for believing in me. Special mention also to the committed team of professionals at MDPublish.com for turning my dream of a book into a reality.

Contents

Introduction

"We restore, repair and make whole those parts which nature has given but which fortune has taken away, not so much that they might delight the eye, but that they may buoy up the spirit."

— **Tagliocozzi**
Plastic surgeon, 1597

Beauty begins with a vision

My philosophy is simple: The key to making patients happy is knowing when to operate, and more importantly, when not to. I often talk my patients out of having cosmetic surgery for various reasons. In my view, if you are not willing to practice sun avoidance and take good care of your skin and your body, surgery is not the answer. Great strides have been made in alternative therapies that effectively reverse the aging process, thereby reserving surgery as a last resort. Throughout this book, you will find discussions about the appropriate roles of topical therapies, treatments, and cosmetic surgery.

The best approach to total rejuvenation is a holistic one that encompasses every aspect of your life from diet, sun exposure, and fitness, to monitoring the flux of your hormones and minding your stress level.

I first became interested in skin care while I was a plastic surgery resident in New York. At that time, most plastic surgeons had not yet embraced the notion that comprehensive skin rejuvenation and maintenance programs could impact surgical results. It was not until the late 1980s that doctors in the cosmetic fields began to emphasize advanced skin and body care and early intervention.

Recognition of the value of advanced skin care is reflected in the recent proliferation of medical spas; they fill a niche between a doctor's office and a luxury resort by offering clients a total experience based on the symbiotic relationship between feeling good and looking good. Aside from traditional spa therapies incorporating hydrotherapy and moisturizing facials, these advanced spas combine the best of science and beauty.

Women and men are flocking to spas not because they are sick but because they want to stay well, feel healthy, and look great. The modern spa concept has evolved to encompass a broad range of wellness services including alternative medicine. I view these spas as a natural extension of the doctor's office. Patients with skin or cosmetic problems may need to see a doctor, an aesthetician, a skincare professional, or all three. Combining medical science with aesthetics benefits everyone — especially my patients.

The biggest trend in aesthetic medicine currently is the integration of organic ingredients with high-tech therapeutic treatments to create significant, long-lasting benefits. Based on this trend, I have developed a special interest in the effects of specific ingredients on the skin, especially before and after surgery. As an aesthetic plastic surgeon, I am trained to view the skin in a complex way. The quality of my patients' skin is crucial to determining their particular surgical outcomes. To that end, I assembled a team of experts to work alongside me in formulating new and improved concepts in skin rejuvenation. The inspiration for these new products and techniques is derived directly from the needs of my patients.

In 1998, we introduced www.TotalSkinCare.com, one of the first comprehensive Web sites to offer medically formulated, nonprescription skin care products. Many of these products were formerly available only through plastic surgeons' or dermatologists' offices, or upscale spas. At TotalSkinCare.com, we offer only the finest, most respected names in skin care, specially selected by doctors and our paramedical skin specialists.

The process of selecting a skin care regimen can be a minefield for the average consumer. Skin rejuvenation products have always been challenging to assess, since there are so many claims and counterclaims from competing manufacturers. I limit my recommendations to products whose effectiveness has been well documented and to those that demonstrate long-term results.

In *Total Rejuvenation*, I focus on the most important aspects of what your skin needs and what it will respond to, just as I do for my own patients. In the following pages, I share my personal insights into the mistakes people make regarding skin care and treatment programs.

Everyone wants to improve his or her skin. It is not an easy task, but if you have the right tools and proper direction from the experts, it is a goal that is within your reach.

— *Barry J. Cohen, MD, FACS*
   Diplomate, American Board of Plastic Surgery

The Science Behind Your Skin

1

"Beauty is the promise of happpiness."

— Henri Stendahl
French writer, 1783-1842

What is beautiful skin? That is a subjective question. Most people would answer by using adjectives like smooth, radiant, glowing, unblemished, evenly pigmented, clean, firm, unlined, and poreless. The keys to achieving these descriptions are prevention and early intervention.

No two people on earth age at exactly the same rate. As we age, our skin goes through a gradual state of change. With each passing year, our skin begins to lose some of its glow, structure, and youthful resiliency. Genetically programmed chronological aging causes biochemical changes in collagen and elastin, the connective tissues that give skin its firmness and elasticity. Everyone's genetic program is individual; loss of skin firmness and elasticity will occur at different rates and times among individuals. As early as our 25th birthday, the skin begins a slow, gradual descent as it starts to become lax. By the age of 60, the skin is visibly sagging. This is especially noticeable on the face, which is subject to the most environmental abuse. The skin thins and loses some of its structure and elasticity and can no longer fight the effects of gravity. A lifetime of pulling by the muscles under the skin and damage from environmental exposure sets the stage for the formation of wrinkles.

Occurring simultaneously with genetically programmed aging is the process of photoaging. Photoaging is the effect of chronic and excessive sun exposure on the skin, and is responsible for as much as 90% of age-associated changes in the skin's appearance such as mottled pigmentation, surface roughness, fine wrinkles that disappear when stretched, brown spots on the hands, and dilated blood vessels. We look at skin aging as the slow accumulation of damage, eventually revealing the symptoms we commonly associate with age. A total skin rejuvenation program takes time and commitment to be effective. Sun exposure and tanning must be effectively eliminated, and a comprehensive program combining state-of-the-art skin care with clinical treatment solutions should be implemented. There is no magic bullet.

Skin Nutrition

The skin is a living organ — the body's largest. It separates the internal environment from the external. Proper nutrition and exercise is important for healthy skin as well as overall good health. Exercise stimulates your metabolism, causes you to sweat, and increases lymphatic drainage, which keeps your skin healthy and clean. Water is an essential skin nutrient. Protein, vitamin C, calcium, and other minerals are a good foundation for any skin care regimen. When nutrients are ingested and absorbed into your bloodstream, they are sure to be delivered to your skin cells. Nutrition has an effect on the mechanisms of aging as a whole. Inhibiting these mechanisms slows down the aging process, including the aging of the skin. Nutrients and foods that benefit your skin also benefit other bodily functions. Vitamins A, B, C, D, E, and K, folic acid, zinc, selenium, and essential fatty acids all contribute to the skin's overall health. They act as antioxidants, scavenging for harmful byproducts in the body and boosting the immune system or promoting healthy cell growth.

Free radicals are the result of oxygen molecules being oxidized, but they can also be created by exposure to various environmental factors, such as smoking and ultraviolet (UV) radiation. Free radicals are known as one of the primary factors that accelerate the aging process. Free radicals are common in all people, and the body can, for the most part, defend itself with antioxidants that are found naturally in the body and that serve as free radical "scavengers." These antioxidants can be used up quickly, which is why taking additional antioxidants in supplement form is useful. Several key antioxidants — selenium, vitamin E, and vitamin C — have been proven to decrease the effect of the sun on the skin and actually prevent further damage.

Selenium

The mineral selenium is necessary to the antioxidant glutathione peroxidase, which helps protect the body from cancers, including skin cancer. Selenium also preserves tissue elasticity, and slows down the aging and hardening of tissues through oxidation. The best dietary sources of selenium include whole grain cereals, seafood, garlic, and eggs. When taken orally in daily supplements of 50 to 200 micrograms, selenium has been shown to offer protection from the sun's rays.

Vitamin E

Vitamin E is the most important antioxidant in the body. It protects cell membranes and prevents damage to membrane-associated enzymes. It can be found in vegetable oils, especially sunflower oil, grains such as wheat germ, brown rice and oats, nuts, dairy products, meats, and margarine. For additional sun protection, individuals may consider taking vitamin E supplements.

Supplementation with 400 milligrams of natural vitamin E per day has been noted to reduce photodamage and wrinkles and to improve skin texture. The best form of vitamin E is its natural form, d-alpha tocopherol.

Vitamin C

Vitamin C is the most abundant antioxidant found naturally in the skin. It is essential for life and is a water-soluble antioxidant that clenches free radicals and regenerates vitamin E. It is commonly found in vegetables and citrus fruits.

Much like vitamin E, vitamin C is important for preventing free radicals from accelerating aging. Even minimal UV exposure can decrease the vitamin C levels in the skin by 30%, while exposure to the ozone of city pollution can decrease that level by as much as 55%. Most people get the recommended daily allowance of vitamin C if they eat more than five servings of fruit, vegetables and juices. Five hundred to 1,000 milligrams of vitamin C are recommended to be taken internally daily. Vitamin C plays an important role in the formation of collagen, which is important for the growth and repair of body tissue cells, gums, blood vessels, bones, and teeth. It is particularly important for smokers to take vitamin C supplements because epidemiological studies have shown that smokers have a significantly lower plasma level of vitamin C compared with nonsmokers. Scientific studies have also shown that vitamins C and E can protect you from skin damage caused by UV exposure.

Beta Carotene

Beta carotene is a pro-vitamin A, which means that once it enters the body, it is converted to vitamin A. Carotenoids, including beta carotene, come in several different forms that are actually better absorbed in a supplement form than from foods. The carotenoids in foods may be difficult for the body to break down. Cooking helps to break them down which helps to increase absorption, but overcooking breaks down the nutrients in the carotenoids themselves. Beta carotene supplements taken in doses of 5,000 IU a day can help in the wound-healing process both before and after surgery, especially in people who take oral steroids like prednisone.

Although overall balanced nutrition is the starting point for staying young and healthy, recent research has placed an emphasis on the role of arginine and zinc in addition to antioxidants.

Arginine

Arginine is an amino acid, one of the building blocks that make up protein, and is responsible for the growth and continued health of bodies, including the skin. It has been linked to enhanced immunity and wound healing and can be found in foods such as fortified oat flakes, cooked oatmeal, wheat germ, cottage cheese, beef, and nuts. The best advice is to get this amino acid through your diet.

Zinc

Zinc is essential for normal pregnancies, responsible for growth and transmission of genetic material. It is also required as an enzyme component of the eyes, liver, kidneys, muscles, and skin. Almost all of our cells contain zinc, with the highest concentration in the bones, prostate glands, and eyes. A zinc deficiency can result in a delayed healing of wounds. Most people get enough zinc from food sources such as lean meats, nuts, legumes, and whole grain products, although too much zinc in the diet can cause toxicity.

External Influences

Just as what we put into our bodies is reflected in our skin, environmental factors play a significant role in how we age. The effects of smoking, alcohol, medications, and stress can be a dull, discolored, and lined complexion that looks older than its years.

Sun exposure. Sun exposure is the single most damaging environmental factor for your skin. Sun-damaged skin looks very disorganized under a microscope, with uneven skin layers that generally result in skin dysfunction.

Smoking. A single puff of a cigarette contains 1 x 1,017 free radicals. This is 100 quadrillion — more than one for every cell in your body. Look at the skin of a smoker: it has a yellow or grayish hue. Smokers are more prone to getting wrinkles and their wrinkles also tend to be deeper. Smoking causes a flood of free radicals to form in the body, which speeds up the aging process. Wrinkles appear sooner — in the early to mid-30s — especially around the mouth and eyes.

Drinking. Alcohol in small amounts has some positive effects on the body. For problem drinkers, the negative effects of alcohol also appear in the skin. If you consume more than one ounce of alcohol per day, you are undermining any effort to fight wrinkles. Alcohol, which is a diuretic, causes blood vessels to dilate and the skin to lose moisture, resulting in dehydration, sagging and a loss of resiliency. Alcohol reduces the body's vitamin absorption rate and slows down the immune system, lessening your natural ability to ward off acne-causing bacteria.

Soap-based products. Everyone has natural oil covering their skin. When this oil is removed by frequent use of drying agents such as soap, the skin becomes dry which can lead to cracking and flaking. Once cracking occurs, the skin is susceptible to inflammation and itching. Harsh detergents tend to have a high pH, which robs the skin of natural lipids and can denature keratins in the skin, causing them to lose function.

Although oral supplements can potentially improve the appearance of visible lines, topically applied agents are required to keep skin moist. In addition to minimizing the effects of environmental factors, effective skin care can build up the structure and elasticity of the skin.

Skin Structure

The skin is composed of two basic layers, the epidermis and the dermis. The epidermis, which is the outer layer, protects us from the environment. The dermis, the inner layer, provides strength and structure to the skin. Although we identify them as separate layers, they comprise one system and what happens to one layer has a direct effect on the other. In order to maximize your rejuvenation results, you cannot ignore what is happening within the dermis or the epidermis. Over time, sun, smoking, stress, disease, and aging alter the structure of the skin, making it sag and lose its luster and suppleness.

The Epidermis

The epidermis is comprised of four main layers that are constantly transitioning upward. In effect, the four layers are actually stages that each cell or keratinocyte passes through on its way to becoming part of the stratum corneum.

The epidermis is the outer layer of the skin. New cells generated by the dermis continually replace this layer. Removal of the epidermis, as in a scrape or burn, reveals an unprotected sensitive dermis underneath. The epidermis serves as a barrier to the outside world, keeping out water, sunlight, germs, heat and cold, dirt, and gases. It also keeps in fluids such as water and blood, and retains minerals, vitamins, hormones, proteins, and heat. The dermis regulates heat for the body by controlling sweat evaporation and dermal blood flow. It protects the body with a tough outer layer to resist friction, abrasion, and pressure.

The complete replacement of the epidermis takes approximately 45 to 74 days, a rate which varies with age. The stratum corneum is fully replaced in about 14 days when we are young, but over age 50, replacement can take as long as 37 days. This delay continues as we age and accounts for the eventual degradation of the skin. In older people (age 80 or more), the skin is quite thin and nearly transparent. The skin is unable to replenish itself quickly enough and becomes frail and easily damaged.

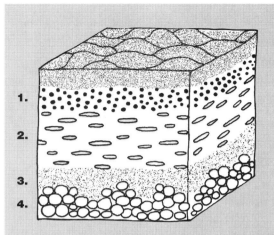

1. Stratum corneum

Where the keratinocytes are cornified becoming corneocytes, which comprise the surface of our skin.

2. Granular layer

Where the cell's nucleus is broken down and keratin fibers form, changing the cell into a keratinocyte.

3. Spinous layer

Where the new cells begin the transformation process, and become unable to divide or grow.

4. Basal layer

A layer of cells that endlessly replicate new cells to replenish the process.

The Dermis

The dermis is the inner layer of skin that contains nerve fibers, blood vessels, sweat and oil glands, and hair follicles. Sweat and oil glands in the dermis protect the outer layer of skin with a thin coating of oil and perspiration. The dermis accounts for more than 90% of the skin mass and for the greatest part of its physical strength. The dermis also contains collagen and elastin, two proteins that are responsible for the structure and elasticity of the skin itself. These proteins are the keys to the aging process.

The dermis has two major layers; the top layer is the papillary layer and the lower layer is the reticular layer. Both of these layers contain the proteins

The Layers of the Dermis

Papillary layer
The outer part of the dermis. It is thin, contains small, loose elastin and collagen fibers, and the lymphatic and blood vessels. The papillary layer is in direct contact with the epidermis.

Reticular layer
Located under the papillary dermis and immediately above the fat layer. It contains most of the connective tissue, has fewer cells, relatively few blood vessels, and dense collagen bundles as well as elastin fibers. It carries most of the physical stress of the skin.

collagen and elastin, but collagen is primarily in the lower layer while elastin is mainly in the upper layer. Collagen is a tough, fibrous protein with a structure that is wound into a triple helix so that the resulting fibers have a high tensile strength. More than 70% of the dry weight of skin is comprised of collagen. Elastin, which comprises only about 0.6% of the dry weight of the skin, has a great influence on how our skin looks and gives skin its resiliency. Fibroblasts are large oval cells responsible for the production of collagen and elastin. They are also located in the dermis, as are glycoaminoglycosans. These complex proteins located on the surface of cells are sometimes referred to as the "glue" that binds the skin.

In theory, photoaging can be prevented. If you could protect your face from the sun all the time, it could remain relatively youthful and wrinkle-free as you age.

Skin Aging

In theory, photoaging can be prevented. If you could protect your face from the sun all the time, it could remain relatively youthful and wrinkle-free as you age. It is critical to start a program of sun protection early in life. It has been estimated that up to 50% of our total UV radiation exposure is acquired by the time we reach 18, and 75% by age 30. Even though the clock for photoaging starts ticking early, we can minimize further changes by practicing sun avoidance. Photoaging steadily develops even with minor UV exposure. The skin does not need to burn (or even turn pink) for slow, permanent damage to take place. Any steps you take to cut down the time you spend outside unprotected will reduce the speed and extent of your eventual photoaging, whenever you begin.

Cellular Function

On a scientific level, aging is a decrease in functional capacity. The metabolism of oxygen, environmental effects and how we treat ourselves all cause damage to the cells that results in aging.

Each cell is like a bubble, a transparent cell membrane that holds a sticky fluid called cytoplasm. The cytoplasm surrounds the three basic structures of the cell: the nucleus, the mitochondria, and the endoplasmic reticule. The nucleus holds DNA, our genetic code and the template from which proteins are made. Antioxidants are our defense against oxidative stress. Some antioxidants are produced by the body and others come from external sources, but we need a constant supply of them to ward off oxidative stress.

The Sun's Effects

The wavelengths of light are measured in nanometers (nm); one nm is one-billionth of a meter. Classifications of light wavelengths include ultraviolet A (UVA), ultraviolet B (UVB), and visible light. The dosage of energy that is absorbed during exposure is the most critical factor in determining the amount of skin damage from the sun. It does not matter how short a time you are exposed if the intensity is high. Shorter wavelengths, such as UVB, have a higher intensity and deliver more energy than the same amount of exposure to longer wavelengths, meaning more damage occurs more quickly. UVA light, which is used in tanning booths, is the prime culprit behind premature aging of the skin.

Wrinkling, sagging, discoloration, and hyperpigmentation are greatly accelerated by sun exposure. We can effectively reverse this damage, but the continuous insult from the sun must be stopped for any treatment to work. Any doctor will caution you that sun protection is mandatory; everyone should wear a broad-spectrum sunblock to shield against both UVA and UVB year-round.

Do's and Don'ts for Glowing Skin

Some of the factors that determine how long your skin will stay glowing include genetics, the condition of your skin, diet and nutrition, your history of sun exposure, smoking and drinking, and your stress level. Preserving a healthy, youthful complexion takes work. A proper skin-care regimen is the all-important first step. Skin rejuvenation is a maintenance process that typically takes six months to generate results. You may be able to see some improvements sooner, particularly in texture and hydration. Be patient — beautiful skin is worth the wait.

In the realm of skin rejuvenation, we are concerned with either hydrating or exfoliating the stratum corneum. Desquamation is the natural shedding of the stratum corneum. The desquamation process involves many enzymes that break down the bonds that hold our corneocytes or skin cells together. One of the main reasons skin sheds is to eliminate damaged cells and cells that are contaminated with bacteria and environmental pollutants and toxins. This process protects and cleanses the skin so that it can respond to its environment appropriately.

Exfoliation

One of the basic methods for improving skin and softening fine wrinkles is exfoliation, the removal of the dried top layer of surface cells. The epidermis, or outer layer of skin, goes through a process of reproduction and maturation. Basal cells at the bottom of the epidermis produce cells that move up through the epidermis. Later hardening of the cells takes place and as new cells come to the surface, the old cells then shed. The cornified layer's function is to act as a barrier, keeping moisture inside the body and foreign substances outside. When these cells remain on the surface, the skin looks dull and flaky.

Methods for exfoliation run from simple scrubs and rejuvenating creams to intensive peeling treatments. Using topical antiaging products in combination with other treatments remains the best approach to treating aging skin. I recommend that most people exfoliate at night on a daily basis.

Research continues to give rise to new and promising antiaging agents. As a plastic surgeon, I look at data with a very critical eye. I am trained to ask product formulators about validation of test methods, and review stability reports to see that the data supports the product's expected shelf life. It is important not to over-sell any ingredients or specific products, since they may produce only subtle visible changes. As long as you have realistic expectations of the kind of improvements you can achieve, cosmeceuticals are an invaluable tool in the treatment of the most common skin concerns — oiliness, dryness, wrinkles, and enlarged pores.

Skin Fitness R~x~

2

"There is certainly no absolute standard of beauty. That precisely is what makes its pursuit so interesting."

— John Kenneth Galbraith
Economist, born 1908

While free radicals have been implicated in the damage that occurs to aging skin, there are other factors, including metabolic imbalances, that prevent aging skin cells from performing repair functions. A skin cream may provide a number of important substances, but it is never enough to ensure optimum skin nutrition. Every cell in the human body needs dozens of nutrients and metabolites. Some, such as vitamins, minerals, and essential amino acids, should come from food sources. Others are produced by a healthy and well-nourished body. No topical product can replace that. Applying a cream enriched with nutrients to the surface of your skin does not ensure that those nutrients actually penetrate into the cellular level. If the molecules are too large, they may just sit there until your next shower. How much of the active ingredients actually gets into your skin cells depends on the skin's condition, the concentration of the ingredients, the technology, and the delivery system, among many other factors. An additional concern is whether agents can be consistently delivered to specific layers of the skin in order to induce a biological effect.

Most people are beginning to practice wise sun protection far earlier in life, which accounts for the dramatic increase of 50 year-olds who look 35. Part of that is also the increased use of good skincare products in recent years. The past 15 years have seen an increasing array of options for skin repair, most notably tretinoin (Retin-A®) and the hydroxy acid family. There is no perfect skin rejuvenation product and no magical therapy that does it all. By judiciously selecting complementary products, you can capitalize on the most effective technology for your individual skin profile. Although they are still not quite like cosmetic surgery in a bottle, we have made great strides.

Cosmeceuticals from A to Z

Key Ingredients

Making good decisions in skin rejuvenation doesn't mean using every product available, or finding one that works "better" than all the rest. It is more sensible to incorporate several active ingredients that work in a complementary fashion and are appropriate for your skin type.

The science of skin care can be baffling. Reading about skin care technology seems like a biochemistry lesson at first. Science is applied to the skin just as it is applied to other vital internal organs. Vitamins can provide many benefits, yet with so many different derivatives, consumers are confused about what ingredients to look for and what products to select. The answer can be found in specific ingredients and how they interact with the mechanisms of aging skin.

Cosmeceuticals are topical cosmetic-pharmaceutical hybrids intended to enhance the health and beauty of skin. Although cosmeceuticals are topically applied, they contain ingredients that influence the biological function of the skin. It is often difficult to determine whether claims about the action or efficacy of cosmeceuticals are valid unless the product has been approved by the FDA or equivalent agency.

There are a host of variables that determine efficiency. I know from clinical research that what works well in the lab may not be feasible in the real world because of packaging issues, problems with shelf life, loss of potency over time, temperature instability, ultraviolet radiation, and exposure to the environment. The active ingredient must be stabilized, delivered to the skin at a therapeutic concentration, and must remain in the skin long enough to exert its biochemical effects. Only when these conditions are met can benefits be achieved.

Each ingredient is derived from a different source, is active in a different way, and produces different results than the next. For example, comparing alpha hydroxy acids (AHAs) and antioxidants is like comparing apples to oranges. However, by incorporating them together into a skin care routine, the skin receives improved synergistic benefits.

Ingredient Checklist

- Must be stable
- Has to penetrate the skin in an active form
- Needs to be delivered in a high enough concentration to be effective
- Has to be used on a consistent basis

Star Performers

There are several helpful active ingredients whose usefulness has been proven in skin rejuvenation. There is also a wide variety of antioxidants, an array of ingredients which play a supporting role and some new, still unproven entries into the rejuvenation scene. Some ingredients may have a place as a stand-alone product or they might be used as part of a multi-step approach. For example, an alpha hydroxy acid peel followed by the application of topical growth factor may increase the penetration of the growth factors, which may reduce inflammation and speed healing. The potential variations and applications are endless, which makes the field of cosmeceutical research particularly exciting.

In aging skin cells, naturally occurring antioxidants are in short supply. Free radicals are left to cause damage to cell membranes, proteins, and DNA, and eventually break down collagen and release chemical mediators that cause inflammation in the skin. It is a combination of these cellular and molecular events that leads to the formation of wrinkles. Many of the compounds currently used in anti-aging skin care products have some antioxidant properties to replace the naturally occurring antioxidants that diminish with age.

Vitamin A

While there are some new agents on the horizon for skin rejuvenation, vitamin A was the first antioxidant to be widely used in skin care. There is significant scientific evidence that substantiates the benefits of topical vitamin A on aging and sun-damaged skin. The synthetic derivatives of vitamin A, called retinoids, are available by prescription only. The ability of these compounds to soften fine lines and wrinkles, lighten pigmentation, and improve overall photodamage makes them the gold standard against which all new ingredients are compared.

Retinoic acid acts as a chemical peeling agent that helps the skin to renew itself more rapidly. The use of retinoids has had a major impact on many skin conditions including acne, rosacea, and photoaging. When used consistently, topical retinoids can be beneficial in preventing as well as in treating photodamage.

R$_x$ Creams

There are currently two prescription-strength formulas approved by the FDA for treating photoaging: Renova® and Avage®. Renova® (Ortho) is a vitamin A cream used for skin rejuvenation. It contains 0.05% or 0.02% tretinoin, the same active ingredient in Retin-A®, and also contains a moisturizing base. The base is made to hydrate mature skin, but the formula is oily enough to flare acne in skin types that are still dealing with oily skin. Tazorac® (prescription-strength tazarotene), which was already FDA approved for treating both psoriasis and acne, has been shown in recent medical studies to rival the results of Renova® in treating photoaging. Under the name of Avage® (Allergan), it is FDA approved for treating aging skin.

Glycolic Acid

Glycolic acid appears to be the most effective of the alpha hydroxy acids for skin rejuvenation because it is the smallest molecule with the greatest penetration. Glycolic acids weaken linkage of cells in the outer layers of dry skin, allowing the normal shedding process to occur. They also increase the flexibility of the outer layer of the skin and may increase the barrier function. Other benefits of glycolic acid include its moisturizing ability, its potential to lighten skin discolorations, and its utility in helping other agents to penetrate the skin more deeply. Medical-strength glycolic acid needs to have a minimum concentration of 8%. This is the baseline where effective results will be achieved.

Bioavailability

Studies have proven that the efficacy of alpha hydroxy acid (AHA) products is directly related to the bioavailability of the AHA. At higher concentrations, mild irritation and peeling may occur. Bioavailability is not always equivalent to the number on the label. The most effective formulas deliver the optimal concentration with the least irritation. Once an acid is mixed into a formula, a question arises as to how much of the acid actually gets delivered to the skin. Neutralizing the acid with a buffer inactivates it, allowing less of the active ingredients to be delivered to the skin. The effects of glycolic acid are concentration dependent. The more acid that gets delivered, the more effective a product will be.

When using AHA-containing products purchased at drug, grocery, or department stores, the percentages are generally negligible. The average over-the-counter AHA level is only 3%. There is a growing trend for product formulators to incorporate higher concentrations into their formulas based on consumer demand.

For maximum results, I recommend a program of in-office peels combined with an at-home glycolic skin care regimen. We start our patients on a lower strength glycolic acid formulation, and as their skin becomes acclimated to this level of therapy, we increase the concentration.

Lactic Acid

One of the hydroxy acids, lactic acid is found naturally in substances such as buttermilk, yogurt, powdered skim milk, sour cream, blackberries, and tomatoes. It is also the substance which builds up in human muscles during exertion, causing muscle pain. It is a natural choice for people who manifest allergies to other hydroxy acids. Lactic acid is a gentle exfoliant and promotes shedding of thickened epidermal skin layer, speeding the natural cell turnover process.

A Word about pH

The natural acid mantle that covers the top layer of your skin is composed of sebum, sweat, and other cell secretions, and acts as a natural defense barrier against skin infections. To stay healthy, skin needs to maintain the proper pH levels and the proper level of acidity.

The pH of a product indicates its acidity. For example, a pH of one or two is very acidic, while a pH of four or five is only lightly acid. A pH of seven is considered neutral. Human skin has a pH between 4.5 and 6. When you wash your face, or even just splash water on it, you remove the natural protective acid mantle from your skin, raising the pH level. Raising the pH of the skin through cleansing alters the skin's natural balance and can be drying or irritating. It may also encourage your skin to age more rapidly.

When a product is "pH balanced" it means that in the formulation, chemical buffers were added so that the product has a constant pH or level of acidity. Generally, skin care products are most effective with a pH of 3.0 or greater.

Kinetin

Kinetin is a naturally occurring growth hormone found in plant and animal DNA that has antioxidant and antiaging properties. Some studies suggest that it may both delay the onset and decrease the effects of aging on skin. The topical formulation is primarily used for its skin rejuvenation effects. In plants, this growth factor helps keep the plant green and healthy. It is formed as a self-defense mechanism against oxidation created by photodamage and helps slow the cellular aging process.

Recent studies indicate that kinetin increases moisture retention, improves fine lines and can lighten sun-induced pigmentation. Kinetin-containing lotions such as Kinerase® and Almay Kinetin are well tolerated, which makes them a good choice for individuals with sensitive skin who are unable to use retinoids and alpha hydroxy acids. These products are purported to produce the same benefits as retinoids without the side effects of peeling and burning. Kinetin-containing products are not acidic so they neither burn nor cause increased photosensitivity.

Kinetin N-6 Furfuryladenine

- Well tolerated
- Non-acid formula
- Non-irritating
- OTC alternative to retinoids

Copper Peptides

First recognized for their ability to enhance wound healing, copper peptides are known to be important in the synthesis of collagen and elastin. Most of the research on copper peptides has been completed in the area of wound healing, but recent studies have demonstrated a favorable response to topically applied copper peptide creams in photo-damaged skin. One of the main advantages of copper is that it is nonirritating and relatively inexpensive compared to other antioxidant creams. Copper peptide has been shown to increase collagen synthesis, aids in the formation of free radical scavengers, and stimulates the skin rejuvenation process. A peptide found naturally in human skin and tissue, GHK (glycyl-L-histidyl-L-lysine), binds copper molecules, allowing them to arrive in an active state where needed. The two most common GHK copper peptides are prezatide copper acetate and copper tripeptide.

Copper peptides help to stimulate collagen and elastin formation, improve skin strength, thicken the dermis, and increase blood vessel formation and oxygenation within the skin. Copper peptide formulas are ideal for sensitive skin, rosacea, or eczema, or for anyone seeking a gentle skin rejuvenation option. Ideally, copper peptide formulas should be used in the morning because they help fight UV rays which may penetrate sunscreen.

Vitamin C (L-Ascorbic Acid)

Vitamin C is technically an AHA (citric acid) but is additionally a potent antioxidant. Ascorbic acid is necessary in the synthesis of collagen. L-ascorbic acid activity requires a very low pH (less than 3.5) to penetrate the skin and to maintain its effectiveness. This can cause some minor tingling upon application. The drier your skin, the more sensitive it may be to the acidity. Studies have shown that vitamin C levels in the skin are depleted after UV irradiation and that vitamin C can improve and normalize the changes caused by prolonged sun exposure. Vitamin C has been used effectively to stimulate collagen repair, thus diminishing some of the effects of photoaging. However, it is very unstable and easily degraded by heat and light, which can make it ineffective. Topical vitamin C can also prevent the damage of prolonged sun exposure.

Vitamin E

Topical natural vitamin E, called d-alpha-tocopherol, reduces chronic UV-induced damage and the production of cancer-causing cells. In addition, topical d-alpha-tocopherol can soothe dry, rough skin. When combined with vitamin C, both vitamins create a highly protective barrier against sun damage.

Alpha Lipoic Acid

Alpha lipoic acid (ALA) is a super-potent fat and water-soluble antioxidant, which makes it different from most other antioxidants available in cosmeceutical vehicles. It is an acidic compound, so high levels can be irritating to the skin. ALA can penetrate skin cells easily through the lipid rich cell membrane and continue to be effective once inside the cell due to its water solubility. ALA has also been shown to exhibit a protective effect on vitamins E and C, thereby boosting naturally occurring antioxidants within the cell. ALA is being touted as a superior antioxidant compound. However, there is still very little data on the effects of alpha lipoic acid on human skin. It is used primarily for its antiinflammatory properties.

Lipoic acid is beneficial for the treatment of pigmentary disorders (see Chapter 3) in much the same way glycolic acid is. It enhances desquamation by allowing superficial, melanin-containing cells to slough off. When lipoic acid is used in conjunction with a tyrosinase-inhibiting agent such as hydroquinone, azelaic acid, or kojic acid, the cells that are sloughed off are replaced by cells that contain less melanin. ALA is available in many different forms and vehicles in concentrations ranging from 1% to 7%. The recommended concentrations for aging skin range from 1% to 4%.

Dimethylaminoethanol (DMAE)

One of the major problems of advanced aging is the sagging of tissues caused by the destruction of the skin's underlying support structure, primarily collagen and elastin. DMAE has been shown to produce a firming effect on the skin. This mechanism may be due to the fact that DMAE functions as a cell membrane stabilizer. Based on early clinical reports, DMAE may be the first topical agent that can help firm sagging skin. Recently, topical formulas containing DMAE have been touted for their ability to improve skin firmness and lift sagging skin, but the mechanism of action in the skin is still unknown. DMAE has been used as a dietary supplement and is associated with improving mental function and enhancing physical performance.

Growth Factors

Growth factors are a new category of compounds being used to treat aging skin. Extracted from cultured epidermal cells, placental cells, human foreskin and even plants, growth factors are compounds that act as chemical messengers between cells, turning on and off a variety of cellular activities. Studies have confirmed an increase in dermal collagen after topically applied growth factors.

Growth factors are a group of proteins that perform a vast array of functions in human growth and development. Each member of the growth factor family binds to a unique receptor. The bound growth factor initiates or, in some cases, blocks cell division. Growth factors work alone and in concert to regulate specific types of cells and tissues.

The earliest products in this category were derived from bovine sources, but growth factor-enriched solutions on the market now are derived from human sources. The growth factors

Common Human Growth Factors

- Transforming Growth Factor-beta (TGF-beta)
- Vascular Endothelial Growth Factor (VEGF)
- Platelet-Derived Growth Factor (PDGF)
- Keratinocyte Growth Factor (KGF)

are contained in liquid compounds derived from the nutrient solutions utilized in the process of creating bioengineered skin tissue. These growth factor extracts contain a number of active compounds, some of which are important in collagen synthesis. New products containing cellular growth factors, used alone or in combination with existing products such as alpha hydroxy acids, are finding a place in skin rejuvenation. The role of solutions containing growth factors in the clinic is evolving.

Spin Traps

Compounds called spin traps are at the cutting edge of cosmeceutical advancements. Known for their ability to bind free radicals, spin traps have been used primarily in the lab setting in the past but are now being studied as therapeutic agents. Spin traps have antioxidant and antiinflammatory properties, and they have been shown to be beneficial in treating inflammatory conditions like rosacea and sunburn. Free radical spin traps combine with reactive free radicals to produce nonreactive free radicals, thus blocking the free radicals from damaging cellular components. Spin traps may emerge as a useful new technology in skin rejuvenation.

Niacin

Niacin is a component of the B vitamin complex whose topical form shows promise as an over-the-counter ingredient useful in antiaging products. One derivative of niacin, nicotinamide, has been shown to improve the ability of the epidermis (the uppermost layer of the skin) to retain moisture. In a recent study, topical nicotinamide was shown to produce softer, smoother skin, less dryness and flakiness, and a reduction of fine lines. The benefits to the skin can be useful for patients with dermatitis, or dry and irritated skin. It is also useful as a treatment for aging skin which frequently becomes dry and flaky with age. Niacinamide, another derivative of niacin, has been shown to be an effective skin lightening agent. It also has anti-inflammatory properties, which makes it a potential treatment for acne and rosacea.

Vitamin K

Vitamin K plays an important role in blood clotting and studies have shown it to be a requisite material to maintain strong bones in the elderly. It can also be used to treat dark circles under the eyes. Dark circles may be hereditary for some people or simply a part of the aging process. When the fat pad beneath the eye begins to thin with age, it can create a sunken look to the under eye area. Studies have shown that sluggishness of blood flow underneath the eyes may also contribute to dark circles. Vitamin K has been found to diminish the appearance of these dark circles, and it can be especially effective when combined with retinol, which has been shown to boost collagen production in the skin. (Occasionally, allergy sufferers who have chronically rubbed the areas under their eyes due to itching and watering may truly change the color of the skin in this region.) Vitamin K has also been studied for its effects on reducing bruising following certain procedures and on speeding healing time after laser treatments and other cosmetic surgery.

Grapeseed Extract

Grapeseed extract contains powerful antioxidants known as oligomeric proanthocyanidins (OPCs) or procyanidins. Pycnogenol from pinebark extract, and constituents of wine, cranberries, green and black teas, black currant, onions, and hawthorn are similar to grapeseed extract in their active ingredients and medicinal uses. The OPCs are reported to possess a broad spectrum of biological, pharmacological and therapeutic activities against free radicals and oxidative stress. Topically, grapeseed extract has been used in cosmetic preparations due to its purported antiaging effects and ability to inhibit enzymes such as collagenase, elastase, and hyaluronidase that are involved in the breakdown of structural components of the skin.

Coenzyme Q10

Coenzyme Q10, called ubiquinone, is a naturally occurring antioxidant that is present in skin. Exposure of the skin to UV light, associated with photoaging, results in a decrease in ubiquinone. In cultured human cells, ubiquinone has been shown to decrease UV radiation-induced oxidative stress and to decrease the activity of certain enzymes that degrade collagen.

Skin Typing

As you might expect, the majority of people classify their skin as "normal." "Combination" skin ranks a close second. "Dry" and "somewhat oily" are about equally common, with "oily" being the least common. Skin type, as categorized by oil secretion, is determined by heredity and classified according to the skin's degree of oiliness or dryness. Generally, skin type correlates with pore size.

Each person has a basic skin type, which can change based on external factors. Your skin type may be affected by factors such as work space, local climate, and season of the year. Dry skin is due to a combination of lack of water and oils in the skin. Even oily skin can lack moisture and be dehydrated. Combination skin features areas which are dry and others which are oily.

Skin Type Grid

Normal skin. Normal skin has an equal balance of water and oil, making it naturally well moisturized. The pores are medium-sized. When you pull the skin away from the bony structure, it springs back to normal position. Lines and wrinkles are appropriate for age.

Oily skin. Oily skin has a coarse texture. Usually, oily areas tend to shine. Oily skin results from overactive oil glands; the oil helps retain dead skin cells in the hair follicles. Pores tend to be larger. The dead skin cells may darken with exposure to the air, forming blackheads. Oily skin types have a tendency to develop acne as teens and overgrown oil glands in the middle and late years.

Dry skin. Dry skin has a rough texture and may become flaky. There are no shiny areas; in fact, the skin looks dull. Pores tend to be smaller because less oil is produced. Without adequate moisture, dry skin can easily become chapped. As dry skin ages, it is more likely than other types to become wrinkled.

Self Test

To determine your skin type, wash your face and wait 30 minutes. Then put a single piece of tissue paper against four key areas of your face: forehead, nose, chin, and cheeks. Oily areas will leave oil residue on the tissue paper.

Know your skin type

Are you mostly oily, dry, normal, sensitive, or combination? If your skin is combination, identify which areas are oily vs. dry.

Know your complexion

Fitzpatrick Classification

I. Very fair skin. ("I never tan, I burn.")

II. Light skin. ("I may tan, but I usually burn.")

III. Light to medium complexion.
("Sometimes I tan, sometimes I burn.")

IV. Medium complexion.
("I usually tan, rarely burn.")

V. Dark complexion. ("I never burn.")

VI. Black complexion. ("I never burn.")

Prioritize your concerns

Do you want preventative maintenance to avoid premature aging? Do you have a skin problem, such as acne, melasma, or rosacea? Are enlarged pores your primary concern? Do you have eye puffiness or under-eye bags? Is your skin sun damaged with wrinkles or fine lines?

Assess your personal habits

Are you a smoker? Did you or do you now spend a great deal of time in the sun? Do you eat a well-balanced diet and get enough exercise? All of these factors will affect how you should care for your skin.

Combination skin. Combination skin is a mixture of dry and oily areas of differing degrees. The T-zone consists of the forehead, nose, and the area around the mouth, including the chin. The percentage of oil glands in this T-shaped area tends to be higher than on the outer cheeks, which makes it more prone to enlarged pores and blackheads. The neck has fewer oil glands and tends to be dry. More people have combination skin than severely dry or oily skin.

Choosing a Regimen That Works

I firmly believe that the basis of all effective skin care regimens should be sunscreen in the morning and a treatment product like a prescription retinoid at night. Every regimen should be altered in special situations and this is only a rough guideline.

Step 1: Cleansing

I encourage my patients to wash their faces with a gentle nondetergent soap that contains moisturizers. The skin should be patted dry and lubricated with a water-based moisturizer to prevent further dehydration. Gentle scrubbing with a mildly abrasive material and a soap that contains salicylic acid can help remove old skin so that new skin can grow. Organic loofahs, sea sponges, and washcloths may harbor bacteria; nonorganic textured sponges do not carry this risk. Some cleansing grains contain pulverized walnut shells and apricot seeds, which can lacerate skin on a microscopic level. Cleansing grains with microbeads don't have sharp edges and remove skin more gently. The rubbing, which should be perpendicular to the wrinkle, mechanically removes the outer layer of dead skin cells. Exfoliation with harsh scrubs can worsen certain conditions, such as sensitive skin or broken blood vessels.

For daily use, mechanical cleansing in the form of cloths or pads can be very effective. These are slightly abrasive, which helps with makeup removal. I also suggest some inexpensive liquid cleansers such as Cetaphil Daily Facial Cleanser, Purpose Gentle Cleansing Wash or Neutrogena Fresh Foaming Face Wash. If you have acne, rosacea, photodamage, or pigmentation problems,

Skin Care Plan

- Wash daily with lukewarm water and limit your time to 15 minutes or less in the bath or shower.
- Avoid using harsh soaps which dry the skin. Use detergent-free cleanser only for the face.
- Limit the use of soap to body areas that develop an odor such as the armpits and feet. Alkaline soaps, especially with deodorant, should be avoided.
- When toweling dry, do not rub the skin. Blot or pat dry so there is still some moisture left on the skin.
- Next, apply a moisturizer to the skin. Concentrate on areas of your skin that become dry. If you have oily skin you can skip this step.
- All areas that are exposed to the sun, especially the face, ears, hands, and back of the neck, should have a moisturizer containing sun block or a sunscreen of SPF 15 minimum applied daily.

I recommend a salicylic acid-based cleansing product used three times a week, such as the Oil-Free Acne Wash by Neutrogena or the Daily Facials Cleansing Cloths with Beta Hydroxy by Olay.

Step 2: Moisturizing

Replacing moisture lost to aging is a prime reason for using face creams. Most commercial face creams are oil-based and work by blocking the release of water from the skin. As we age, skin loses the ability to attract moisture and becomes dehydrated. At this point, aging skin needs to be replenished with a natural moisturizer complex in order to attract and retain water. Moisturizing is like a savings plan with the benefits only showing after time. Moisture is essential for skin to look younger, healthier, and smoother. Moisture gets stored in skin cells between fatty layers and as the skin ages, these cells find it harder to retain that moisture thus leaving skin feeling dry, rough, brittle, and more prone to flaking and cracking.

Most people need to moisturize once or twice a day, but oily skin may only require a light moisturizer applied once daily. When choosing a moisturizer, take into account your age, lifestyle, skin type, and what you are hoping to achieve. Moisturizing products alone are not going to turn back the clock.

Moisturizers are needed where your skin feels dry. For anyone with dry skin or for those who live in a dry climate, an additional moisturizer may be necessary. Moisturizers prevent water from evaporating from the skin by providing a protective coating of emollients.

Be wary of over-moisturizing your face. It can be tempting to keep adding layers, but too much moisturizer can block pores. Many sunscreen products contain sufficient moisturizers on their own. If you are layering moisturizer, foundation, and sunscreen, consider combining them by choosing a foundation with built-in moisture or a face cream with added sun protection.

Common Emollients

- Mineral oil
- Petrolatum
- Cholesterol
- Lanolin
- Dimethicone/cyclomethicone
- Almond oil
- Jojoba oil
- Avocado oil
- Sesame oil
- Sunflower oil
- Grapeseed oil

Moisturizers that bind water, thereby retaining it on the skin surface are called humectants.

Widely Used Humecants

- Glycerin (glycerol)
- Propylene glycol
- Sorbitol
- Hyaluronic acid
- Lecithin
- Urea
- Lactic acid
- Collagen
- Elastin
- Ceramide

Step 3: Sunscreen

Sunscreen. Chemical agent that blocks or absorbs ultraviolet light, making the wavelengths incapable of causing damage.

Sunblock. Agent that acts as a physical barrier to prevent sunlight from reaching the surface of the skin.

There is tremendous confusion concerning the differences between various formulations of sunscreen versus sunblock. The ideal sunscreen is one that will provide you with the necessary level of protection for your skin type, degree of sun exposure and sun sensitivity. The safest rule to follow is to generously apply an SPF 15 broad-spectrum sunscreen every two hours. Most people do use sunscreen today; however, they do not use nearly enough to provide adequate coverage. The higher a product's sun protection factor rating, the stronger and longer its effects. However, the SPF index only addresses UVB rays, and there is no standard measurement for protection against UVA rays. Parsol 1789, zinc oxide, and titanium dioxide are the key UVA blockers.

Both men and women who get intense sun exposure during outdoor sports or boating should use more complete coverage, meaning a sunblock of SPF 30 or higher. Waterproof lotions have an oil base which is thicker and heavier and may clog pores. When a product is labeled "water resistant," it means that it provides the stated level of SPF after water-resistance testing has been done for a specified length of time. Even water-resistant formulas

Buy products with adequate labeling; for example, a list of ingredients and the name and address of the manufacturer or distributor in case you have a problem. Stop using any product immediately if you experience adverse reactions, including stinging, redness, itching, burning, pain, bleeding, or increased sun sensitivity.

will need to be reapplied after swimming, exercise, or sweating. For oily skin, stick with oil-free formulas that won't make you look and feel shiny or cause you to break out. Also look for waterproof sunscreens that will not run into the eyes.

Step 4: Treatment

Any prescription retinoid brand can be used, including Tazarac, Differin®, Avage, Retin-A Micro®, Avita®, Retin-A, or Renova. Creams are usually preferred by women. Gels are often more suitable for younger women and men. For excessively dry skin or for those who live in an arid climate, Renova may be best. Begin by using a pea-size amount applied to the entire face every third night for two weeks. Then apply the retinoid of choice every other night for two weeks. If it is well tolerated, you can start applying it every night. Some people will never be able to move beyond the every third night regimen but will still benefit from using it in this fashion.

If you cannot tolerate prescription retinoids, over-the-counter retinol-containing preparations can be used instead. Retinols may not be as effective or work as quickly as prescription formulas, but there is clinical evidence that they can make visible improvements in the skin.

Making Adjustments

The products and practices which kept your skin looking beautiful in your 20s will not necessarily work as well when you enter your 30s, 40s and beyond. Like your lifestyle and your wardrobe, your skin care regimen needs to be updated as times passes. Don't wait until you turn 40 to start caring for your skin. Beginning early can delay the formation of lines, wrinkles, and pigment changes.

The skin is remarkably resilient; however, skin becomes normalized to the environmental conditions it routinely faces. Drastic changes in the environment require the skin to make adjustments. For example, traveling to a dry climate or the sudden dryness of winter often results in itchy, dry patches until the skin responds by increasing oil production to reduce the water loss. Similarly, changing cleansers or moisturizing products may also tilt the skin's balance in relation to the environment.

In Your 20s

The most important thing you can do for your skin, no matter what your age, is to wear sunscreen every day. This is particularly true when you are young. It's important to realize that you receive more than 80% of your lifetime sun damage before the age of 18. As you progress into

What to Use in Your 20s

Wear a broad-spectrum sunscreen with an SPF rating of 15 or higher. A mild cleanser with acne-fighting ingredients (such as salicylic acid or sulfur) can prevent future outbreaks. Stay away from heavy creams and oily products that clog pores — young skin has sufficient natural moisture.

your 20s, you may have less acne than in your teens, but women in particular may still struggle with hormonal acne along the jaw line and chin.

In your 20s, skin cells regenerate at top speed, giving you a radiant look. Collagen and elastin, the fibers that give skin its plumped-up look and elasticity, are in optimal shape. The damaging effects of photoaging have yet to appear.

In Your 30s

In your 30s, you may notice that your skin is less oily and may even seem flaky and dry in places. Your skin may appear to be in flux – oily one minute, dry the next. Acne breakouts are still common. You may notice that your skin looks different in your 30s, even though you may not be able to pinpoint exactly why. First, cell regeneration has already started to slow, making skin look a bit dull. Second, collagen and elastin aren't being produced as rapidly, so you may start developing fine lines.

What to Use in Your 30s

Find products that don't irritate your skin and that contain antioxidants such as vitamins C and E, and beta-carotene, which repair and prevent further damage. Continue to use non-comedonegenic products to avoid occasional breakouts. Begin using a daily moisturizer with SPF 15 under makeup, and an eye cream at bedtime.

In Your 40s

Healthy aging occurs differently for everyone. As collagen production slows down, skin also loses firmness and elasticity. These and other normal aspects of skin aging such as wrinkling, appearance of small blood vessels, mottling, and age spots are intensified by accumulated damage from past sun exposure, smoking, drinking, and poor diet. Forty-year-old skin may occasionally break out in blemishes because of premenstrual hormone surges or perimenopausal hormone fluctuations. Oil production in the skin diminishes, and it is important to keep moisturizing. At this age, wrinkles around the mouth and eyes will become apparent.

What to Use in Your 40s

A well-balanced skin care regimen should include protection and treatment, as well as adequate moisturization. Begin using more potent alpha hydroxy acid products to help remove the dead outer layers of skin. Tretinoin at night can help soften fine lines and age spots.

In Your 50s

As you age, the skin begins to lose its plumpness and tone. Individuals may also notice more irregular pigmentation and age spots. This is an excellent time to have a skin examination, since a suspicious-looking spot may be an actinic keratosis, a precursor to skin cancer. You also may notice a persistent redness across your cheeks and nose that may be rosacea, a common and treatable condition that begins as a tendency to flush or blush easily, and can progress to persistent redness in the center of the face that may gradually involve the cheeks, forehead, chin, and nose.

What to Use in Your 50s

An active skincare regimen with a combination of antioxidants for skin firming and rejuvenating effects such as copper peptides or kinetin is critical. Hydration becomes increasingly important due to moisture loss. Don't over-cleanse, which can dry out thinning, aging skin. Bleaching agents can be useful to reduce age spots and blotchiness.

In Your 60s and Beyond

At this age, the skin may have numerous wrinkles and deep creases, and have a pale appearance with very lax or loose skin. Pigment is lost in the skin and lips. Age spots appear more readily.

What to Use in Your 60s and Beyond

Skin care becomes less effective as you age, and more invasive treatments will be needed. Lasers are extremely effective for treating deeper wrinkles and severe sun damage or irregular pigmentation. Skin is thinner and more susceptible to sun damage, so a higher SPF is recommended daily. At this stage, cosmetic surgery will be necessary to make a significant change in facial aging.

Specialist Skin Solutions

3

"Personal beauty is a greater recommendation than any letter of reference."

— Aristotle
Greek philosopher, 384-322 BCE

How to Treat Common Problems

There are certain stages and times in everyone's life when their skin looks and feels great, and other times when it disappoints them. Many factors influence these changes, including stress and how well you are taking care of your skin at that particular moment. My team has received thousands of queries, e-mails, and letters from women and men of all ages across the country, with surprisingly similar concerns about acne, hyperpigmentation, and sensitive skin.

Acne treatments are perhaps the fastest-growing segment of the skin care realm today, second only to antiwrinkle products and treatments. Hyperpigmentation is another common concern which can be even more problematic in darker or bronze skin types. The other principal area of concern is skin sensitivities, such as allergic, reactive, or easily irritated skin. In the following sections, I have addressed all of these key skin care issues and offer solutions that can help you navigate through the myriad of products and treatments on the market. If your problem is mild to moderate, you may be able to see a big difference just by using the recommended products for your skin type. If your problem is moderate to severe, you may need to seek professional medical advice for the best solution.

Acne Remedies

Acne is the most common skin disorder in the United States, affecting 85% of the population at some point in their lives. Most of us see a pimple, and think acne. It's easy to be fooled into thinking you have acne when it could be another skin condition entirely. For example, dermatitis can show up on the lower face and chin in the form of red, inflamed blisters. Blackheads are flat, darkened spots, which are the result of pores becoming plugged with oil or sebum and dead skin cells. The dark center of a blackhead is dried oil and dead skin cells in the openings of hair follicles. Blackheads commonly appear on the face, (especially around the T-zone), on the bridge of the nose, and on the back, chest, shoulders, and upper arms.

The best treatments for blackheads address their cause: the processes of oil production and skin cell turnover. Effective treatment serves to dry the skin and slow oil production, and to remove skin debris so that it cannot clog the pores.

The goal of acne therapy is to eliminate existing lesions and prevent the formation of new ones. Acne is treated by interfering with its developmental process. Acne occurs when androgen hormones cause sebaceous glands to grow and produce excess sebum. The skin cells of the follicle lining shed quickly and in clumps. These cells and increased sebum output are likely to cause clogged pores, which become comedones. Finally, *P. acnes* bacteria which is normally present on the skin invades the clogged follicle and begins to multiply rapidly. The result is acne in all of its forms.

By treating blackheads when they first appear, you can avoid some of the more difficult problems associated with more advanced forms of acne.

Acne by Definition

Blackheads

"Open comedones" which are formed when dead skin cells and sebum are tightly packed inside a follicle whose walls have broken. If the plug enlarges and pops out of the duct, it's referred to as a blackhead. The skin cells and oil give it a dirty appearance that simply won't wash away.

Whiteheads

"Closed comedones" where the plug stays below the surface of the skin so that the follicle wall does not break. Whiteheads are formed on or under the skin.

Papules

Red, raised bumps or inflamed lesions that occur when the oily material inside the follicle ruptures into the surrounding skin.

Pustules

Similar to papules but slightly more inflamed with visible pus.

Cysts

A severe form of inflammatory acne, cysts are closed hard sacs that can be painful, and are usually treated with prescription drugs.

I commonly prescribe retinoids for acneic skin, and they can make a tremendous difference in the overall appearance of the skin by speeding cell turnover and slowing down oil production. Two or more acne products are sometimes used to treat different acne causes.

What Do Acne Treatments Do?
- Reduce sebum production
- Reduce *P. acnes* bacteria
- Normalize the shedding of skin cells

Extraction of comedones should only be performed by a professional under sterile conditions, and usually only when comedones have not responded to other treatment. While it might be tempting to self-treat blackheads, picking or squeezing blackheads sideways may break the oil gland and aggravate the acne. This can result in inflammation and possible scarring. With appropriate treatment, acne should go away without squeezing.

Regular washing twice daily with a salicylic acid cleanser temporarily helps to remove debris and surface oil that can clog the pores. Toners or astringents containing salicylic acid can also be helpful for oily skin. Avoiding foundations and other products containing oils is also helpful. Some water-based foundations have oil in them, so choose oil-free, water-based products or a flesh-tinted acne lotion containing benzoyl peroxide, salicylic acid, or sulfur. Other treatments for blackheads are alpha hydroxy acid and salicylic acid peels which are used as a first defense to prevent cells from building up and clogging pores. Microdermabrasion is also a useful modality to remove surface blackheads. Pore strips can dislodge debris, but the adhesives of pore strips can cause irritation and increase the production of new blackheads.

Over-the-Counter Acne Formulas

Benzoyl peroxide. A mainstay of over-the-counter acne treatment and a medication commonly prescribed to treat mild forms of acne. Benzoyl peroxide was the first agent proven to be effective in the treatment of mild acne. Its antiacne effects are believed to be antibacterial with an accompanying decrease in some constituents of sebum. Benzoyl peroxide is available over the counter in a lotion or a gel. Its principal side effect is to cause excessive dryness of the skin. Salicylic acid helps to correct the abnormal shedding of cells. For milder acne, salicylic acid helps to unclog pores to resolve and prevent new lesions. Like benzoyl peroxide, it must be used continuously since pores will clog if discontinued. Sulfur, in combination with other agents like alcohol, salicylic acid, and resorcinol, is also found in over-the-counter acne preparations. Resorcinol is used together with sulfur as well.

Topical Antibiotics

Topical antibiotics are often used in combination with other topical agents. Azelaic acid cream, a naturally occurring acid, has been adapted for acne treatment. Erythromycin is active against a broad spectrum of bacteria. A combination erythromycin and benzoyl peroxide commonly maximizes the effects of two antimicrobial agents and reduces skin oiliness. Clindamycin and tetracycline are also used topically, as well as sodium sulfonamide lotion which is available for the treatment of acne and for reduction of inflammatory lesions.

Topical Retinoids

Retinoids are very potent antiacne medications because they normalize abnormal growth and reduce dead cell residue in the sebaceous follicle. Retinoids are available in both topical and systemic forms. The systemic form, isotretinoin or Accutane®, is usually reserved for acne that is resistant to other treatments. The most common side effects of topical retinoids are redness, dryness, peeling, and itching of skin in the areas of retinoid application.

The topical natural and synthetic retinoids currently available as acne medications in the United States are:

Tretinoin. Influences skin cell growth and death cycles. Topical tretinoin is available as a cream, gel, or solution.

Adapalene. A synthetic retinoid applied as a gel or cream. It has potent retinoid and antiinflammatory activity.

Tazarotene. A synthetic retinoid applied as a gel or cream. It acts on the follicular cell cycle by a biochemical pathway different from that of tretinoin.

Isotretinoin

The gold standard of acne therapy, particularly for cystic acne, is isotretinoin (Accutane). Isotretinoin, a synthetic retinoid, is usually reserved for the most severe forms of cystic acne and acne that is resistant to other medications. It can be very effective in treating most forms of acne. Remission for many months to many years is possible. The most common side effect of isotretinoin is dryness of the skin and mucous membranes. Other, less common, side effects include nausea and vomiting, bone and joint pain, headache, thinning hair, depression, and changes in blood and liver enzyme profiles which are monitored in regular follow-up examinations. For most people, the side effects are tolerable. Women who are planning a pregnancy, are pregnant, or are nursing must not use isotretinoin as it can produce severe birth defects in children.

Oral Medications

Broad-spectrum antibiotics have been a mainstay for moderate to severe and persistent acne for many years. The antiacne activity of oral antibiotics appears to include physiologic effects in the sebaceous follicle as well as reduction of bacterial populations in the follicle. Oral tetracycline has a long history in the treatment of acne, and remains one of the most widely used oral antibiotics. Long-term, low-dose tetracycline therapy may be continued for many months to maintain suppression of acne. Higher doses may be prescribed for very severe acne, with regular monitoring for side effects. Oral erythromycin is an alternative to tetracycline that is safe for use in pregnant women. Oral minocycline and doxycycline are synthetically derived from tetracycline and both have a long history of use in the treatment of acne.

Hormonal Therapies

Androgenic hormones are known to have physiologic effects on sebaceous follicles that promote the development of acne. The purpose of hormonal therapy is to block or lessen acne-promoting effects of androgenic hormones. Estrogen is a feminine hormone that counteracts effects of androgenic hormones and decreases sebum secretion in the sebaceous follicles. Estrogen-containing oral contraceptives are prescribed more frequently than estrogen alone for acne. The effects of estrogen are balanced by other hormonal constituents of oral contraceptives. Hormonal therapy may be a treatment of choice for women whose acne does not respond to other medications. The antiandrogen spironolactone reduces sebum production and improves acne in some patients, and may be used along with an oral contraceptive. Some birth control pills have a combination of ethinyl estradiol, a synthetic estrogen, and norgestimate, a progestin. Ortho Tri-Cyclen® decreases the hormone levels that contribute to the development of acne-producing agents, thus attacking the cause of the acne. Yasmin® is a new birth control pill with dual-property progestin and drospirenone which is similar to spironolactone.

Light Treatments

The latest treatment for acne involves the use of laser and intense pulsed light (IPL) systems to destroy the bacteria that cause acne without drugs. New devices emit a narrow band spectrum of intense light directly onto the skin. Light rays convert a substance produced by acne bacteria into an acne-killing compound. Other forms of noninvasive laser treatments deliver energy down to the oil-producing centers in the sebaceous glands to destroy these oil reservoirs without harming the outer layers of the skin. These lasers may work for cystic acne as an alternative to oral and topical medications. Treatments can take from eight to 15 minutes, and may be repeated as needed, once or twice per week for up to eight weeks. In many cases, acne can be controlled for several months at a time. Another benefit is that results may be seen after one treatment instead of eight to 12 weeks with medications. Light therapy can also speed the healing of active lesions, reduce inflammation and improve or prevent acne scars.

Pigment Problem Solvers

When you're young, they're called freckles. As you get older, they're called age spots. Hyperpigmentation simply means an excess of pigment in the skin. If you feel like your complexion is being punished by unsightly brown patches that never seem to go away, you are not alone. Pigmented skin can be difficult to treat, but new options continue to be introduced. State-of-the-art treatment involves combination therapy of topical formulas alongside more aggressive medical treatments and maintenance for best results. The key to managing hyperpigmentation is long-term, total sun avoidance.

Melasma is Greek for "black spot." When it is associated with pregnancy, it is also called "chloasma," or the mask of pregnancy. It is a form of pigmentation on the face sometimes mistaken for a suntan that appears around the cheeks, forehead, upper lip, nose, chin, and jaw line. It can also show up on the forearms, but this is quite rare. Although melasma is most common in women of childbearing age, you don't have to be pregnant or even be a

The key to managing hyperpigmentation is long-term, total sun avoidance.

woman to have it. It is also found in older women who did not have it during their pregnancies, and up to 10% of cases are found in dark-skinned men.

There is no known cure for melasma. In many cases associated with pregnancy, the discoloration fades away after delivery, but may persist indefinitely. The good news is that there are treatments available that can minimize dark patches and keep them at bay. Successful treatment usually begins with the trio of sunblock, bleaching creams, and time.

Melasma tends to darken in summer after sun exposure, and fade in winter when the sun is less strong. This happens because the skin's pigment, melanin, absorbs the energy of the sun's ultraviolet rays in order to protect the skin from overexposure. Tanning occurs as a result, causing dark areas to get even darker. Melasma occurs more frequently in light brown or bronze skin types from regions of the world with intense sun exposure.

As with many beauty concerns, genetics plays a major role in melasma. More than 30% of sufferers have a family history of melasma. Skin inflammations from allergic reactions, or waxing of facial hair (especially above the lip), can also be a trigger. Some medications, such as the antibiotics tetracycline and minocycline and some antiseizure and antimalarial drugs, can also cause melasma.

The first step in the treatment of hyperpigmentation is to determine the cause. A complete medical history and a proper physical examination including an evaluation of the skin should be performed. Diagnostic tests, including thyroid function tests and skin biopsies, may be appropriate. The next step is to eliminate the cause, if possible. For example, if the cause is the medication you are taking, discontinuing it may result in a clearing, but melasma is not always readily treatable. Hyperpigmentation in pregnancy occurs in about 90% of women, mostly due to hormonal changes that are aggravated by sun exposure. It is the result of an overabundant production of melanin in the epidermis. The reasons for this overproduction are associated with sun exposure, injury, infection, and pregnancy.

There Are Two Basic Types of Pigment Production

Constitutive pigment. The base melanin that forms the natural skin color.

Facultative pigment. The enhancement of melanin production by melanocytes, in response to sun exposure (as in tanning.) Facultative pigment is reversible, which is why tans fade with time.

Melanocytes are the cells in the epidermis that produce melanin. They respond to sunlight by producing more melanin to protect the keratinocytes (one of the main reasons for melanin production). Melanosomes form a shield over the nucleus of the living keratinocyte cells to prevent solar radiation damage. Ultraviolet light also causes an inflammation of the skin. The long-term effects of solar radiation will cause pigment to pool from leaking melanocytes. This phenomenon produces age spots. In this case, the melanocyte has been damaged by ultraviolet exposure and needs to be repaired.

With injury or infection, a red papule is formed that eventually turns into a hyperpigmented spot.

No treatment will be effective if you are still tanning. Tanning reverses the treatment process and encourages repigmentation of the skin.

This is due to increased melanocyte activity, which produces more melanin in the affected area. This increased melanocyte activity is in response to inflammation. In a normal situation, when the inflammation subsides, the resulting hyperpigmentation sloughs off as the cell moves to the top of the epidermis.

Tyrosinase is an enzyme that determines just how much melanin is produced. The majority of products available to treat hyperpigmentation inhibit tyrosinase in one way or another. The most well-known agent is hydroquinone, which is still widely considered the most effective skin lightening agent. It works by blocking the action of tyrosinase in the formation of melanin. It can be used to retard or stop production of melanin in many conditions, such as melasma or postinflammatory hyperpigmentation. An uncommon side effect of hydroquinone is a disorder called exogenous ochronosis, which is a progressive darkening of the area. Hydroquinone use should be discontinued if no improvements occur within four to six months due to the potential risks of long-term use. It is currently banned in Europe and some Asian countries.

Major Causes of Pigment Irregularities

- Pregnancy
- Oral contraceptive use
- Genetic factors
- Sun exposure

Product Name	Company	Active Ingredient
Lustra AF, Alustra, Lustra Cream	Medicis	Hydroquinone 4%
Glyquin, Glyquin XM Cream	Valeant	Hydroquinone 4%
Claripel Cream	Stiefel	Hydroquinone 4%
Alphaquin HP Cream	Stratus	Hydroquinone 4%
Solaquin Forte, Eldoquin Forte Cream	Valeant	Hydroquinone 4%
Melanex Solution	Ortho Neutrogena	Hydroquinone 3%
Tri-Luma Cream	Galderma	Hydroquinone 4%, Tretinoin 0.05%, Fluocinolone acetonide 0.01%
Solage Solution	Galderma	Mequinol 2%, Tretinoin 0.01%

Most skin lightening agents work better in tandem than on their own. Lightening agents such as kojic acid are often combined with other ingredients like azelaic acid, glycolic acids, lactic acid, retinol, ascorbic acid, and botanical lighteners.

Following are several agents that have lightening effects on the skin:

Kojic acid. Kojic acid is derived from various fungal and organic plant materials. It helps reduce melanin formation, and has been shown to be statistically equivalent to hydroquinone without the toxic side effects. Additionally, it scavenges free radicals that are released from cells and acts synergistically with magnesium ascorbyl phosphate (see below) to inhibit tyrosinase activity and defend further against free radicals. Kojic acid, like hydroquinone, can also be combined with a variety of other ingredients, including hydroquinone, to help hasten improvement.

Glycolic acid. The most common alpha hydroxy acids (AHAs) used in cosmeceutical formulations are glycolic acid and lactic acid. Glycolic acid can reduce pigmentation and is often used in combination with other skin lightening agents. Glycolic acid is a wonderful base to apply prior to a bleaching agent as it helps draw the bleach into the skin. Several prescription hydroquinone products such as Lustra® (Medicis) and Glyquin® (Valeant) include glycolic acid to aid in penetration and help shed pigment.

Arbutin. Arbutin is found in high concentrations in plants capable of surviving extreme and sustained dehydration. This ingredient inhibits melanin synthesis.

Methyl gentisate. This plant-derived lightening agent is less irritating than hydroquinone and is known to be a powerful tyrosinase inhibitor.

Magnesium ascorbyl phosphate. Magnesium ascorbyl phosphate is a highly stable derivative of ascorbic acid that is converted directly to ascorbic acid in the skin and demonstrates a longer effective duration. It is thought to retain its potency longer than ascorbic acid delivered topically and has a longer shelf life. A 10% concentration of MagC® can suppress melanin formation and acts synergistically with kojic acid to inhibit tyrosinase activity and defend against free radicals.

Mulberry. Sohakuhi or mulberry extract is obtained from the dried skin of mulberry root found throughout Japan. Sohakuhi has been credited with many healing functions and is known for its antiinflammatory and emollient qualities. Mulberry contains phenylflavonoids, which inhibit the activation of tyrosinase.

Bearberry. *Arctostaphylos uvaursi* or bearberry extract has been shown to inhibit melanin production in melanocytes by reducing tyrosinase activity.

Azelaic acid. Naturally occurring azelaic acid is derived from *Pityrosporum ovale*, which is a fungus. Azelaic acid works by inhibiting melanocytes.

Skin lightening is not a quick process. Depending on how dark the area is compared with your normal skin tone, it can take six months to one year to see significant results. Nonprescription lightening creams can go only so far in improving the appearance of melasma. If you are seeking more dramatic improvement, you may have to look to more invasive remedies including glycolic peels, trichloracetic acid (TCA) peels, microdermabrasion, and intense pulsed light treatments, which are the most common methods used to even out skin pigment. These

The primary treatments for hyperpigmentation are an effective ultraviolet A/ultraviolet B sunscreen, a wide-brimmed hat and topical hydroquinone.

treatments tend to be done in a series to get the best long-term results. More intensive treatments tend to be riskier for darker skin types. None should be administered without first using topical bleaching creams. If your skin is prone to hyperpigmentation, this regimen should be followed on an ongoing basis. Sun protection and pretreatment with skin-lightening agents can be useful before any procedure is performed. It should be resumed shortly after re-epithelialization of the skin for prevention and treatment of postinflammatory hyperpigmentation.

Bronze Skin Types

People with darker skin have different complexion issues. The term "bronze skin" includes African American, Asian, and Latino skin types. These skin types are pigment protected so they don't burn as easily as fair complexions, but they are at greater risk for discoloration and melasma. On the Fitzpatrick Skin Scale of I to VI, skin types III and higher have special needs that are not always adequately addressed by the cosmetics and skin care treatments that are commercially available.

An African American or Asian woman at age 50 who has been exposed to the sun will typically have better facial elasticity and look younger than a blue-eyed, blonde European of the same age who has also experienced sun exposure. Delayed wrinkling is related to higher melanin production that provides natural sun protection. The downside is that bronze skin tends to darken before it burns, and can develop chronic hyperpigmentation earlier.

In my practice, the major concern for African American or dark-brown to black-skinned people is discoloration. Postinflammatory hyperpigmentation is a widespread problem. People with darker skin tones often experience discoloration from a variety of causes such as acne, insect bites, scratches, eczema, chicken pox scars, abrasions, or overexposure to the sun. Picking the skin has a tendency to leave deep scars and discoloration that usually appears darker than the rest of the skin. Typical problem areas for discoloration are the joints (ie, knees, elbows, etc.) and eyelid area. This is further complicated by the fact that darker skin types do not always respond well to resurfacing treatments or procedures that can be used to lighten pigmented areas.

Other special concerns include ingrown hairs or razor bumps that are caused by excessively close shaving of curly hair. These can occur on the face, underarms, and bikini area. Keloids and hypertrophic scars are also more of a risk in darker skin types. Fortunately, hypertrophic scars that are raised and pink are far more common than true keloids. The good news is that compared with fair skin types, people with darker and thicker skin are less inclined to need antiaging treatments such as wrinkle fillers, BOTOX® injections, and laser resurfacing.

Black skin. Black skin can be quite sensitive, discolors quickly, and scars easily because of the more active melanocytes. It is much more sensitive to the sun's harmful rays than most people assume, which is a primary cause of the discoloration. Ashy complexions frequently make black skin appear blotchy. Shine from excess oil is also a common problem.

Asian skin. Asian skin can range in complexion from very fair to darker olive shades with yellow undertones, and from extremely dry to exceptionally oily. The higher concentration of pigmentation a person has, the easier they scar and discolor. Yellow-tinted skin has fairly active pigmentation, which makes it very susceptible to sun damage, scarring, and discoloration. More than any other ethnic skin type, Asian skin is the most transparent and soft, which leads to magnification of every spot and scar.

Latino skin. Olive or Latino skin types have the firmest skin of the bronze spectrum. Firm skin can both protect you from deep scarring but may also cause many problems for your complexion. In Latino skin, overactive sebaceous glands bring excess oil to the skin's surface, causing enlarged pores, oily T-zones, and blackheads. Tough skin is frequently the cause of ingrown hairs and dark spots from breakouts.

Skin Sensitivities

Sensitive skin is quite common and means different things to different people. Although clinically sensitive skin is rare, many people experience skin irritations from specific ingredients. At one time or another, your skin may be sensitive; sensitivity can occur in all skin types and in all age groups, and in men as well as women. Some of us are born with sensitive skin, which tends to be hyperactive or easily reactive. Sometimes our environment seems to be making our skin feel sensitive.

Wind, cold, or very hot weather can remove many of the natural humectants that are found in the skin. Dry skin exacerbates any sensitivities you may already have. If your skin feels dry, tight, and itchy, it will be more prone to reactions. People with sensitive skin should realize that anything that damages the skin barrier in the environment can predispose them to developing red, itchy skin. Sensitive, dry or mature skin suffers the most from overexposure to the effects of the environment such as sun, wind, pollution and cold. Fair, thin, and delicate complexions are also at risk for skin cancer, rosacea, and broken capillaries. In some cases, skin becomes more sensitive as time passes due to these effects along with a decreased barrier function.

True sensitive skin types need special care and products that won't exacerbate allergies and reactions. It can be tricky to select products that will minimize potential irritation and breakouts. Limiting the amount of ingredients you use whenever possible is critical. Whether you have truly sensitive skin or just experience frequent skin irritations, select fragrance-free formulas to avoid unnecessary side effects. An increased awareness of specialty products designed for sensitive skin types will make it easier to manage your reactions and keep skin healthy and glowing.

The key is to find out what you are sensitive to and try to avoid it. Reactions can occur as the result of an allergic response of the skin to environmental allergens such as food or inhalants. Remember, factors such as genetic predisposition, climate, and

Don't be too anxious to try every new product on the market. Once you find a skincare regimen that works for you and keeps your sensitive skin under control, stick with it.

exposure to environmental irritants play a role in skin sensitivity. Itching is a common complaint, and scratching can cause bacterial infections. Contact dermatitis may be caused by a primary chemical irritant or by an allergen, like cosmetics, chemicals, and skin care. Continuing use of causative agents may perpetuate skin irritation, so if you experience a skin reaction, first attempt to figure out what caused it, wash it off immediately, and discontinue its use.

When you are sensitive to a variety of ingredients, it becomes harder to find products that do not cause reactions. Don't be too anxious to try every new product on the market. Once you find a skincare regimen that works for you and keeps your sensitive skin under control, stick with it. Sensitive skin requires avoidance of all irritants that can cause inflammation such as soaps, detergents, fragrances, colorants, and alcohol.

Signs of Sensitive Skin

- Reddening
- Tightness
- Scaling
- Stinging
- Breakouts
- Rashes
- Dryness
- Itching
- Flaking
- Blushing

Sensitive skin also reacts to the way it is treated. Although the skin is remarkably robust, harsh treatment over time can lead to increasingly sensitive skin. If you are too aggressive with your skin care regimen, you may aggravate reactive skin. Even though your skin is delicate, you still need to exfoliate to keep skin healthy and glowing. Dry sensitive skin doesn't lack oil; it lacks water and is dehydrated. Light textured, oil-free moisturizers should be applied when the skin is wet after bathing to trap the water in the skin. A humidifier in the bedroom will also help hydrate the skin. Gentle cleansing with a detergent-free formula that does not strip skin of its natural moisture, combined with mild exfoliation twice a week, can rebalance skin. Irritated skin breaks down elasticity and may increase premature aging if you do not take care of it properly.

When the barrier function is weakened, the skin's natural defenses can be compromised and irritants like pollution and UV rays can easily penetrate. Sensitive skin needs extra protection to repair the symptoms which can result when the epidermis has been exposed to irritants.

To reverse the effects of environmental damage and protect the skin from future damage, sun protection is essential. For sensitive skin, it should only contain physical sunscreen ingredients like zinc oxide or titanium dioxide. Unlike chemical sunscreen agents that absorb UV rays, it is impossible to be allergic to physical sunscreen ingredients since they deflect the rays rather than absorb them.

Fragrance is the number one cause of cosmetic sensitivity. According to studies, 1-12% of all people will develop a reaction to a skincare ingedient.

Tips for Reactive Skin

Use products that contain no more than 10 ingredients
The fewer ingredients in a product, the less likely it is to cause a reaction.

Use silicone-based foundations
Choose only liquid foundations with a silicone base that won't cause acne and have a low incidence of skin irritation.

Choose powder when possible
Powder cosmetics are good for removing shine. They have few preservatives and other ingredients that can cause irritation. This means powder cosmetics are less likely than their liquid counterparts to cause problems for women with sensitive skin.

Avoid waterproof cosmetics
Waterproof cosmetics require a solvent to remove them which also removes the oily barrier that can leave skin exposed to potential irritants and cause breakouts.

Throw out old cosmetics
Keep track of cosmetic expiration dates and throw out any items that may have become contaminated. Wash makeup brushes and sponges regularly since they can harbor germs that aggravate sensitive skin.

Your Wrinkle-Free Future

4

"The art of healing comes from nature, not from the physician. Therefore, the physician must start from nature, with an open mind."

—Paracelsus
Swiss physician, 1493-1541

Over the past five years, many of our patients have asked us to recommend skin rejuvenation treatments that can improve wrinkled, blotchy, rough, or sun-damaged skin. Many are not interested in surgery, but rather a more modest, less costly improvement in their skin quality.

Fine lines are due to the breakdown of collagen and elastin fibers over time and are exacerbated by the sun damage we accumulate over the years. Deep wrinkles are typically associated with the build-up of musculature far below the skin's surface. Over time, the use of facial expression muscles will thicken the muscle, just like building a bicep. Deep wrinkle lines may be present on a persistent basis (static wrinkles seen with the face at rest) or may be seen only when those muscles are used (dynamic wrinkles). For example, some people's crow's feet are only obvious when they smile because their cheeks come up, or their frown lines may be evident only when they frown.

Therapy for wrinkles addresses many issues; some are preventative, others are restorative. A characteristic of sun-damaged skin is the degradation of the supporting structures caused by reduced collagen synthesis. The key to maintaining your skin is to keep it taught, with good structure and elasticity. Cosmetic surgery, such as a face-lift, is most effective for deep wrinkles and sagging skin in the lower face, somewhat effective in the middle face, and not effective in the upper face. Cosmetic surgery does not address the other two important factors to younger looking skin: structure and elasticity. A plastic surgeon can, however, reset the clock to a new starting point and help you control your future.

Crinkle-type wrinkles

Fine wrinkles formed around folded skin generally seen in the elderly and people with sun damage.

Glyphic wrinkle

A crisscross pattern that makes a diamond shape usually found on the cheeks, neck, and hands.

Deep wrinkles

A major line or deep grooves that are usually fairly long and straight.

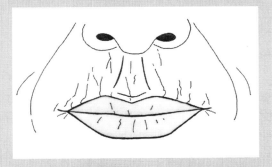

Crinkle and Deep Wrinkles

Fat

As you turn the corner to your 30s and 40s, one of the first signs of aging is the loss of the soft, round, cherubic fullness of the face. We tend to gain weight as we get older. As the natural fat of your face changes shape, hollows start to show up around the eyelids, the middle of the cheeks, and around the mouth. The fatty layer on the backs of the hands, the neck, and face becomes noticeably thinner. This leads to more noticeable blood vessels on the back of the hands.

With aging, the little fat pad under the chin and the pouches along the jaw line start to expand. Fat pad atrophy below the eyes exacerbates the appearance of dark circles, and the overall thinning of the skin allows for increased fragility. The atrophy of the soft tissues of the face fat may also exacerbate some of the deeper wrinkling changes along the jaw line and around the mouth. The thing to remember about fat is that you usually don't have enough where you need it, and almost always have too much where you don't.

Muscle

Fat is found below the dermal layer, followed by muscle. Deep wrinkles are due to the building of muscles in areas of overused facial expressions, such as smiling or frowning. The same can be said of the deep lines that form around the mouth, sometimes called smoker's lines. Chronic puckering of the mouth, particularly if there is additional sun damage, may lead to the formation of deep creases and folds. These will require different therapy than treatments for finer lines associated with damage within the dermis.

Nonsurgical Age Management

Skin rejuvenation is not about looking 18 when you're 80. Rather, it is about choosing a reasonable approach to caring for your skin, keeping it looking fresh and healthy, and making the most of what science and technology offer.

There is a wide array of nonsurgical treatments available that can improve your appearance, soften lines and wrinkles, plump facial contours, and minimize skin conditions like acne, rosacea, and hyperpigmentation. These treatments can be considered as alternatives to cosmetic surgery, or as adjuncts that can enhance and maintain the results of surgery.

To put the skin rejuvenation spectrum in the simplest terms: lifts lift, fillers fill, lasers and peels resurface, and Botulinum toxin paralyzes muscles. Each method has its own purpose and one does not do the job of the other. In addition, each category of technique complements the other well.

My philosophy advocates preventing wrinkles, rather than waiting to correct them once they have appeared. I recommend that my patients begin with smaller, less-invasive procedures and earlier surgery, especially for younger patients. Not everyone wants to have a face-lift, even if there will ultimately be a benefit from surgery to correct laxity and sagging. Many patients prefer to concentrate on nonsurgical, minimally invasive procedures combined with active skin care to forestall the need for a lift later in life.

The Beauty of Botulinum Toxin

The advent of Botulinum toxin (BOTOX®)for cosmetic uses is widely considered to have revolutionized the field of cosmetic medicine over the past decade. Botulinum toxin was originally used to treat eye spasms and central nervous system disorders. Since the late 1980s, it has been used for cosmetic purposes as well as medical therapies.

What Can BOTOX® Do for You?

Botulinum toxin A, a purified protein made from botulism bacteria, binds to nerve endings, preventing the release of chemical transmitters that activate muscles. When injected into specific areas of the face, it paralyzes the small muscles that cause frown lines, crow's feet, and other wrinkles. Treatment with Botulinum toxin decreases local muscle activity, thereby preventing the appearance of "dynamic" wrinkles that are caused by repeated facial expressions. The toxin acts on the junctions between nerves and muscles, preventing the release of a chemical messenger called acetylcholine from the nerve endings.

Tiny amounts are injected into a specific facial muscle so only the targeted impulse of that muscle will be blocked, causing a local relaxation. It acts as a muscle blockade to immobilize the underlying cause of the unwanted lines (muscle contractions), thereby preventing wrinkle formation. Since the muscle can no longer make the offending facial expression, the lines gradually smooth out from disuse and new creases are prevented from forming. Other muscles that are not treated are not affected.

The procedure usually only takes 15 to 30 minutes. First, the skin may be treated with a topical anesthetic cream or gel, if requested. A thin, fine-gauge needle is then used to inject the Botulinum toxin into the skin and muscle, as determined by the doctor. Some physicians use a needle connected to an electromyography (EMG) recorder to guide them to target the most active part of the muscle. Crow's feet are treated with three or more injections on the side of the face close to the outer eye area or orbital rim. Forehead creases are typically treated with 10 to 16 small injections, to weaken rather than paralyze the forehead muscles.

There are actually several strains of Botulinum toxin, but the most commonly used form has to be reconstituted with normal saline before use. BOTOX Cosmetic® received approval for cosmetic use from the FDA in the spring of 2002 for glabellar creases. Approval for another Botulinum toxin type A called Dysport® is still pending from the FDA. Botulinum toxin Type B was introduced more recently. This type comes as a preformulated liquid that does not require a diluting agent. Compared with Type A, it has a longer shelf life (up to two years), requires a larger dose, works somewhat faster, but is also slightly more painful when injected.

Botulinum toxin is considered to be most effective when administered around the eyes and forehead, but other areas of the face and neck can be treated. The effects of Botulinum toxin treatment are not permanent and are reversible. It takes two to 10 days to get the full effect. In most cases, the treatment lasts for four to six months. Some studies have indicated that results can last longer between treatments after multiple treatments. This is theoretically due to the treated muscles' ongoing atrophy or shrinkage from persistent disuse.

Every person responds differently to treatment with Botulinum toxin. Some treated sites last longer than others. Typically, the forehead frowning area lasts the longest, whereas areas around the mouth will not last as long.

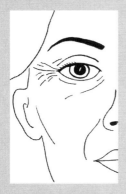

- Lines at the bridge of the nose
- Crow's feet or squint lines (pictured)
- Horizontal forehead lines
- Muscle bands on the neck
- Uneven eyebrows
- "Popply" or "cobblestone" chin
- Chin creases
- Drooping corners of the mouth
- Upper lip lines

Where BOTOX Ends and Fillers Take Over

Botulinum toxin may not be as effective on lines that are not entirely caused by the action of a muscle, ie, the nasal labial folds that are formed by a combination of muscle action and the weight of sagging skin. Some areas cannot be treated because the muscles are needed for expression and important functions such as eating, kissing, and opening the eyes.

For deeper wrinkles, a combination of Botulinum toxin and a filler, such as fat or hyaluronic acid gel, may be recommended. Since the advent of Botulinum toxin in facial rejuvenation, fillers are used less frequently for the forehead and around the eyes. If the creases between the brows are very deep, a filler may be used to smooth it, but Botulinum toxin is usually the first course of treatment. In general, static wrinkles are better treated by fillers, and dynamic wrinkles are better treated by Botulinum toxin. Exceptions to this rule make the use of these products an art as well as a science.

Although there is some discomfort involved with any injections, there is virtually no pain after filler injections. The treatment can sometimes cause a brief headache and bruising can occur at the injection site. Applying ice packs over the treated site before and after the injections can reduce the discomfort, swelling and bruising. You can apply camouflage makeup if needed, and resume regular activities immediately after treatment.

Filling Choices

Soft tissue fillers are substances injected or implanted under the skin. They are used to plump up or contour the soft tissues, and soften wrinkles, furrows, scars and hollows in the face. There are numerous filling substances on the market today, including bovine or cow collagen, human collagen, hyaluronic acid gel, liquid silicone, fat, and polymer implants. The wide array of choices in filling materials makes this area of cosmetic medicine controversial.

The duration of dermal fillers is variable and depends upon the formulation of the material, how deeply it is injected, how much is used, and upon the severity of the wrinkles or folds to be treated. Most dermal fillers are only temporarily effective, so repeat treatments will be needed every three to six months on average. There may be bruising and swelling following any dermal filler treatment. Itching and mild discomfort are not uncommon. Asymmetries, hardening and lumps are also potential complications. Some substances such as bovine collagen require pretreatment testing for allergic reactions. Although less than 3% of the population is allergic to bovine collagen, an allergic reaction may cause itching, hives, redness, and prolonged swelling. Topical anesthetic agents are often used for numbing, and a dental or lip block may be needed for very sensitive areas like the lips and around the mouth.

All doctors have their favorite fillers, and most use several different types. Not every filling substance is right for every face or function, and I like to use a variety of fillers that are suitable for different purposes. Generally, thicker substances are best for deeper creases and for recontouring areas like cheek hollows and lips. Thinner substances work better for fine lines and superficial wrinkles, or in areas where the skin is thin such as around the eyelids and the lip lines.

Each filler is injected in a unique manner, and there is a learning curve to achieve an optimum result. I prefer to have my patients return in two to three weeks after treatment to check their results and refine treated areas as needed.

The Rejuvenating Effects of Fat Grafting

Fat is perhaps the most widespread material used as a filling substance in facial rejuvenation. The fat injected into facial areas comes from your own body, so there is no chance of an allergic reaction. Fat can be used in higher volumes than most other injectable materials and can be used to create a fuller, more youthful appearance by reestablishing pleasing contours. Injections of fat into the deep layers of facial tissue can soften the angular, thin appearance that often accompanies aging. Fat is the first choice when injections of volumes greater than 10cc are needed.

The procedure is a two-step process that usually requires several treatments. Using a small cannula, the fat is harvested from your body, typically from the abdomen, thighs or hips. After it is extracted, it is placed in a centrifuge or allowed to sit for a period of time to separate the fat from surrounding tissues. The fat is then packed into a syringe ready to be injected. Because fat molecules tend to be larger than other injectable materials, it is usually injected more deeply and with a larger-gauge needle. Significant volumes (50cc up to 100cc) can be used over the entire face at one stage. Fat can be particularly useful around the mouth, hollows around eyelids, cheeks, depressions, scars, lips, and in the hands.

Fat injections have a variable lifespan and much of the fat may be absorbed within six months. The fat is slowly absorbed by the body, although the amount of absorption depends on many factors and is hard to predict. Typically, more than half of the fat used in injectable treatments is absorbed within six months of the procedure, although it may last longer. Almost all patients will perma-nently retain some of the injected fat. Follow-up treatments are usually necessary. Your fat can be kept frozen for up to a year, which enables addi-tional corrections to be made.

Putting fullness back into hollows and sunken areas softens the changes associated with aging. Fat works best as a volume filler for deeper creases and folds, not for fine lines. Fat is layered below the skin

If you are not comfortable with the idea of having a foreign substance injected or implanted into your folds and creases, your own fat offers the safest option.

to create a supportive structure in the face, and when this technique is done in stages, it allows for a gradual improvement over time without a long recovery. Fat transfer is also a wonderful complement to all forms of cosmetic surgery, and new techniques can actually make it last longer.

Human Collagen

Filling agents can be derived from human tissues, either your own or products obtained from cadaver tissue through tissue banks. Donor suitability is typically determined according to the standards of the American Association of Tissue Banks (ATB) and the FDA. Cadaver collagen must meet criteria established for extensive testing for human immunodeficiency virus antibody (anti-HIV 1-2), Hepatitis B surface antigen (HBsAG), Hepatitis B core antibody (HBcAB), Hepatitis C antibody (antiHCV), human T-lymphotropic virus type I antibody (antiHTLV-1), and rapid plasma reagin (RPR) for syphilis.

A human tissue filler that received approval in March 2003 is now marketed under the names CosmoDerm® and CosmoPlast® (Inamed Corp.) It contains human collagen that has been purified from a single fibroblast cell culture. This product contains 0.3% lidocaine, so additional local anesthesia is usually not required. No skin test is required because it is made from human tissue rather than from an animal source. CosmoDerm and CosmoPlast are injected just below the surface of the skin to fill in superficial lines and wrinkles and to define the border of the lips.

CosmoDerm and CosmoPlast work much the

same way as bovine or cow collagen do, but will not last as long as some other fillers on the market. Typically, CosmoDerm and CosmoPlast last for two to four months.

Hyaluronic Acid Gels: The Next Frontier

Hyaluronic acid gels have been widely used in Europe, Canada, and South America for the treatment of facial wrinkles and for lip augmentation. Most forms are a clear, transparent, and viscous fluid, free from animal proteins. Hyaluronic acid is a natural polysaccharide that occurs as an important structural element in the skin and in subcutaneous and connective tissues, as well as in the synovial tissue and fluid. Its normal function in the body is to bind water and to lubricate moving parts like joints.

Hyaluronic acid has an identical form in all living organisms. Therefore, in its pure form it is highly biocompatible and requires no pretreatment allergy testing. The source of the material can be from avian protein, or from a nonanimal bacterial fermentation process.

The most common areas for treatment are the nasolabial folds (creases from the nose to mouth), the nasomental creases (corners of the mouth), and around the lips, as well as cheek and chin contours. Since there is no anesthetic supplied in the syringe, some pain relief is needed to keep the patient comfortable, especially in the lip area, which tends to be quite sensitive. Aside from expected temporary redness/puffiness for the first day or two, there are few complications and longevity of six to nine months has been reported.

Of the commercially available fillers, Restylane has had the most anticipated arrival in the U.S.

Of the commercially available fillers, Restylane® has had the most anticipated arrival in the United States. Restylane (Q-Med/Medicis) received FDA approval in 2003, and Hylaform® (Inamed) is expected to be available in 2004.

The Truth about Long-Lasting Fillers

Semipermanent and permanent fillers typically contain synthetic components that do not get broken down by the body. They are considered permanent because the particles cannot be removed, or "semipermanent" because the particles are suspended in a substance that gets absorbed in three to six months. The term "permanent" can be somewhat misleading. As the aging process continues, you will need additional treatments.

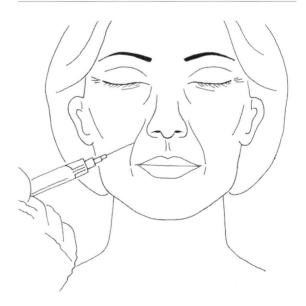

Filling Treatment: Nasolabial Folds

ArteFill.® A semipermanent filler made of 75% percent bovine collagen and 25% polymethyl-methacrylate microspheres (PMMA) which are carbon-based polymers. PMMA has been used in dental work, hip prostheses, and bone cement. The product is mixed with lidocaine to numb the area to be injected. Over three months, the collagen fibers get absorbed, leaving the PMMA behind. These particles are too large to be broken down, and remain in the area permanently. ArteFill is tunneled under the skin with a needle, massaged and molded to fill the area to be treated. ArteFill can be used for acne scars, nasolabial folds, and for filling depressions such as sunken cheeks. Possible complications include lumping, inflammation, granulomas or localized hardening, rash, and the migration of the microspheres into other areas.

Radiance.™ Composed of synthetic calcium hydroxyl apatite, this new filler has been used in the body for multiple applications including cheek and chin implants. Because synthetic calcium hydroxyl apatite is composed of calcium and phosphate ions that occur naturally in the body, Radiance is biocompatible. It is injected into the face and adds volume through microspheres that are suspended in polysaccharide carriers until encapsulation occurs. Calcium hydroxyl apatite has been used for years for other medical purposes in both injectable and solid implant forms.

The particles are in a gel carrier made up of cellulose, glycerin, and purified water. As with any long-term filling agent, there is a possibility of a foreign body reaction which can cause lumps or granulomas, as well as migration. Radiance can last as long as two to four years.

Sculptra.® Based on a substance called polylactic acid (PLA) which has been used in suture materials for years, Sculptra is injected to stimulate production of the body's own collagen within the line or wrinkle, making the skin appear smoother and firmer. The substance is nonallergenic and typically three treatment sessions are recommended for results that can last two years or longer. Widely used in Europe, at the time of printing, Sculptra is entering clinical trials in the United States for approval.

Injectable liquid silicone. Not all forms of silicone are created equal. They vary by degree of purity, and "noninjectable" grade silicone has been problematic when used to treat facial lines. The form making a comeback in the United States is sterile, purified, medical injectable-grade silicone. The newest method of injection is referred to as the "microdroplet" technique, which has the advantage of causing fewer hard lumps than previous variations. Liquid silicone is only approved by the FDA for ophthalmic uses, so applying it for cosmetic purposes is considered an "off label" use of an approved product. Injectable silicone may be beneficial in acne scars and nasal, lip, and chin defects. Silicone is considered permanent, and is difficult to remove if it migrates or causes granulomas or hard lumps.

Long-Term Results

Recovery time will depend on the extent of the treatment and how much material is injected. Most people experience some swelling and redness for the first 24 to 48 hours. When large amounts of any substance are injected into the face, swelling may last from several days to one week. Most injectable fillers have short recovery periods and patients can return to work the same day or the next day. Some people swell more than others and bruising is common, but can be covered with camouflage makeup as needed. In more extensive procedures such as fat injections into multiple areas, local anesthesia or light sedation may be required.

Safety Issues

There are now approximately 70 fillers available commercially worldwide. New dermal fillers continue to be subjected to clinical investigation, and products with a high incidence of reactions and complications have difficulty getting FDA approval. Europe, South America, and other parts of the world have less stringent criteria and fillers are often approved for medical and cosmetic use based on unsubstantiated clinical data. Many products are used in the cosmetic field even though they may not have FDA approval for a specific cosmetic indication. This does not constitute an illegal use of an approved substance. A physician may obtain access to an unapproved drug by participating in a clinical study as an investigator. In some cases, "off label" use means that the drug or filler is approved for a use other than facial wrinkles. For example, Botulinum toxin type A only recently received FDA approval for the application of facial glabellar wrinkles, although it has been widely used for cosmetic purposes since the late 1980s.

Great Lips

Full lips exude sexiness in most cultures. Pouty, sultry lips are highly desired by both men and women. They have become a fashion statement, and celebrities with enhanced lips greatly influence the trend worldwide. Lip enhancement is the single biggest use for dermal fillers, second only to nasal labial folds (nose to mouth lines). Done well, naturally and with a safe filling substance, the results can be wonderful. It is a treatment that spans all ages.

Whether you have always had thin lips, or you want to return your lips to the shape and fullness they had when you were younger, a lip augmentation procedure may provide you with the look you're seeking. A good injector knows just how to make a beautiful lip shape, while maintaining the natural line and contour. It's not just about injecting a filler into the lips to make them bigger; it's a matter of achieving a good shape with natural lines which suit that particular woman.

Like breasts, every pair of lips is different. Some women just need their top lip done. Most women benefit from the top and a little bit on the bottom lip to balance them out. The filtrum (the two points that rest from the nose to the top lip) can also be injected if they are flattened in shape. We often recommend enhancing the lips with micropigmentation to make them appear fuller. There is an art to lip enhancement, and not every injector can create great lips.

If you're not happy with the way your lips were injected the first time, you should go back for a touch-up and explain what you really want.

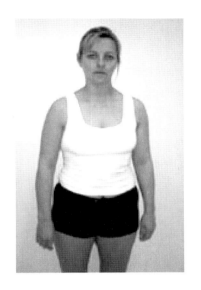
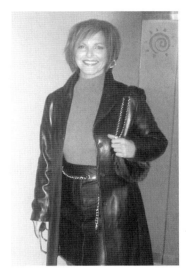

**Makeover—Tummy Tuck/
Liposuction of Abdomen, Thigh,
Neck/Complete Rhinoplasty/
Botox to Face**

Left, preop; right, postop.
26-year old female.

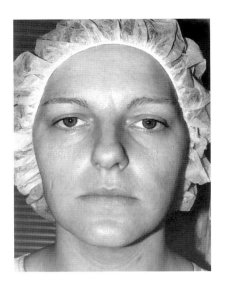 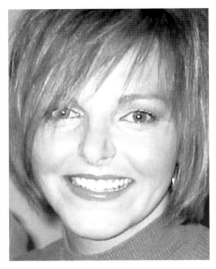

**Rhinoplasty/Liposuction
of the Chin**

Left, preop; right, postop.
26-year old female.

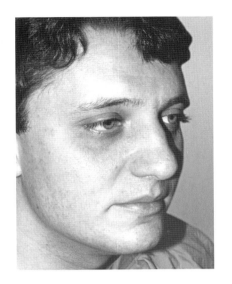 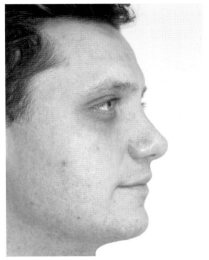

Rhinoplasty

Left, preop; right, postop.

30-year old male.

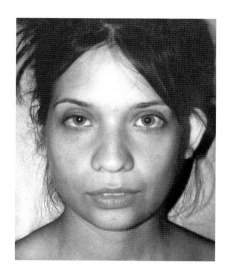 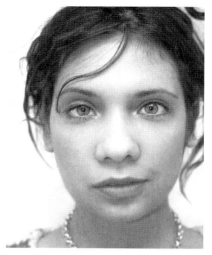

Rhinoplasty/Otoplasty

Left, preop; right, postop.
22-year old female.

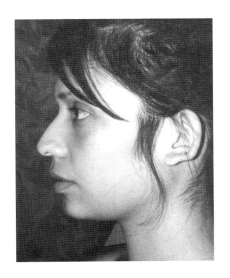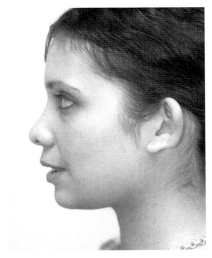

Rhinoplasty

Left, preop; right, postop.

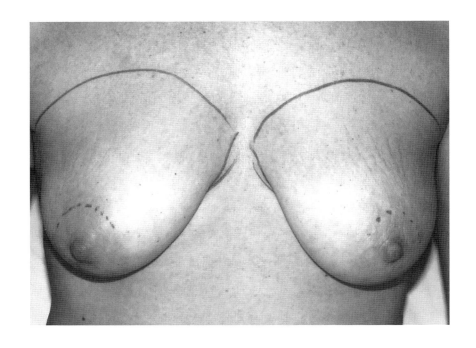

Breast Augmentation/Lift

This page, sagging breasts, preop; facing page, postop, breast lift/augmentation with high profile submuscular saline implants. 41-year old female.

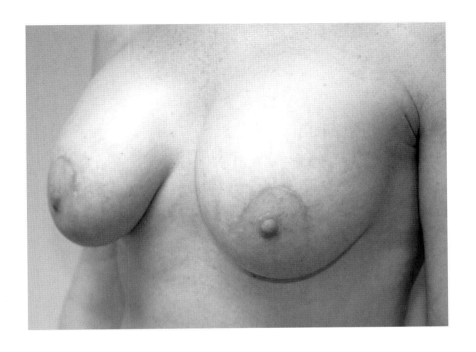

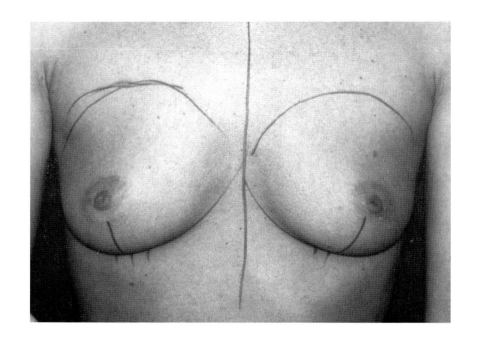

Breast Augmentation

This page, preop; facing page, postop, with submuscular
low profile smooth saline implants.
43-year old female.

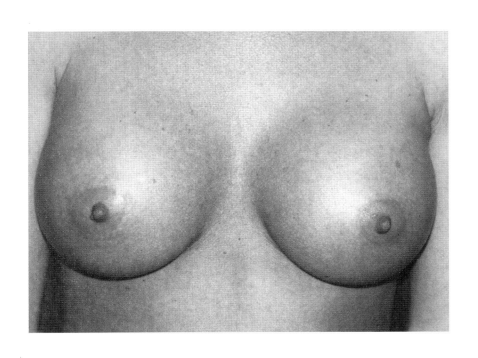

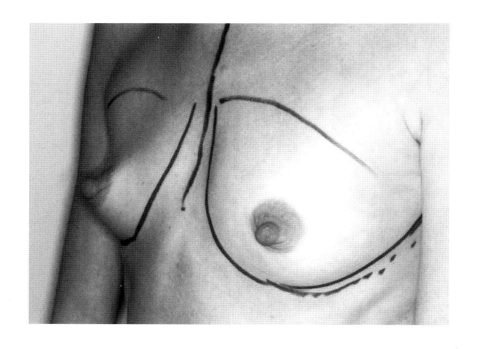

Breast Augmentation

This page, preop; facing page,
postop, with submuscular high
profile saline implants.
33-year old female.

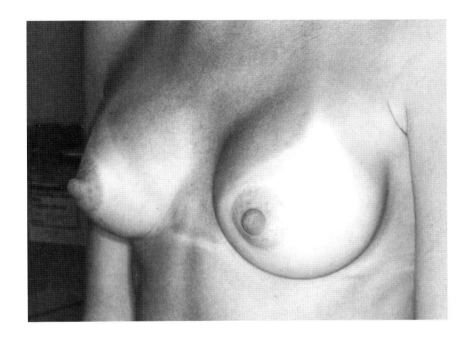

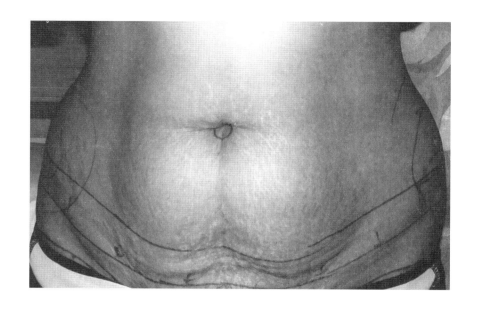

Tummy Tuck

*This page, preop; facing page,
postop, full tummy tuck, liposuction
of abdomen and flanks.
50-year old feamle.*

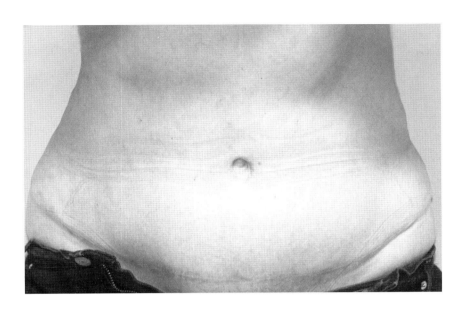

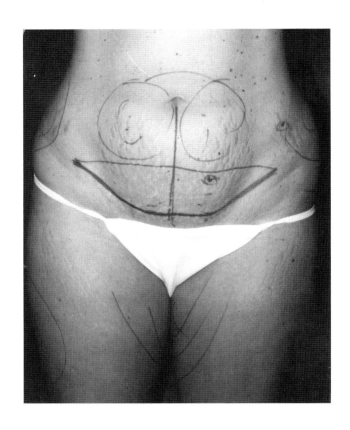

Mini Tummy Tuck/ Thigh Liposuction

This page, preop; facing page, postop.
35-year old female.

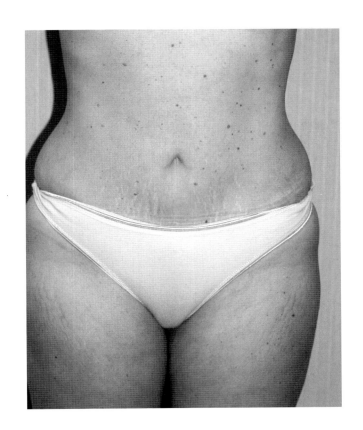

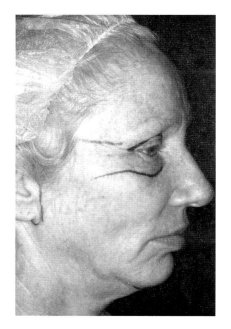 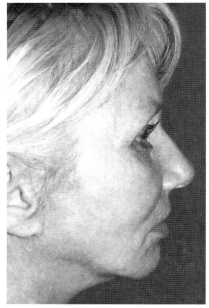

Face-Lift/Eyelid Lift/Brow Lift

Left, preop; right, postop.

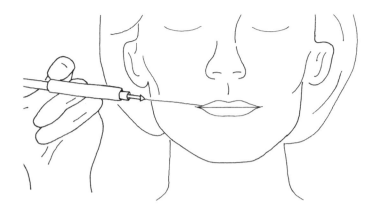

Filling Treatment: Lip Enhancement

Communication is important because there is more than one technique to use and many filling agents that produce different results.

Temporary Lip Plumpers

The most popular substances like Restylane and Perlane® may last from four months to up to one year, depending on the quantity injected, where it is placed, and your lip shape and size. Perlane lasts longer in the lips than Restylane. Zyplast® and CosmoPlast last three or four months in the lips. Anything injected into the lips will not remain as long as in less dynamic areas of the face, because the lips are in constant motion. Fat injections generally work well. All of these will need to be retreated eventually.

When lips are overdone or badly done, the descriptions that come to mind are "trout pout," "duck lips" and "sausage-like." Lips should always pass the kiss test, that is, feeling and appearing soft, luscious, and natural.

Surgical Enhancements

The positive results of lip enhancement are rounder, fuller, more youthful contours to the lips. Lipstick stays on better and the lip line looks beautiful. As we age, our lips thin out and the pigment fades. If you start out with thin lips, by your 40s, they seem to disappear. Women with thin lips will need constant maintenance to get a good result. Women with fuller lips when they are younger need less material injected and fewer, less frequent treatments.

I rarely recommend long-term filling substances for the lips. The possible complications from permanent and semipermanent fillers with synthetic particles include lumps, unevenness, infection, persistent swelling, pustules, hardening, and tightening of the lips. In many cases, if these problems do not clear up on their own, the only remedy is to make an incision and cut out the material causing the problem. This can lead to swelling, bruising, and more scar tissue formation. With temporary substances, you are guaranteed to have your natural lips return to normal when the product gets broken down and resorbed.

I have never been pleased with the results of permanent lip enhancement techniques. I honestly do not think they look natural. One of these techniques, cheiloplasty, involves an incision made at the vermillion border or upper lip line. Another technique, called a lip lift, involves making an incision at the bottom of the nose to raise the lip. This works well if there is a long distance between the tip of the nose and the upper lip. Older people will often see a lengthening of this area above the lips. This operation will shorten that distance, but the scar is permanent and can be quite noticeable on

some people. Permanent implants like Gore-Tex®
and variations have a high rate of extrusion and
infection which have made their popularity decline
sharply. Some surgeons use other natural graft materials such as fascia (the substance that covers the
muscle fibers) or dermis. These can result in scar tissue formation which can make opening your mouth
and smiling difficult.

The skin of the lips is thin and unforgiving. Less is
more when it comes to lip treatments — you can
always go bigger. Once you have surgery and make
a scar, you are effectively stuck with the results since
these are difficult to correct surgically. I often advise
patients to have something temporary done first. If
they like the effect, but insist on something more permanent, I might suggest trying fat transfer. In my
opinion, the younger you start, the more cautious
you should be in considering long-term risks.

The Art of the Peel

Chemical peels vary according to their active ingredients, their strength, their pH, and how long the
solution remains on the skin. Different types of
peeling agents penetrate to different levels of the
skin and, consequently produce varying results.
They are all similar in that they involve applying a
chemical solution to remove damaged outer layers of
skin so that newer layers can replace the old ones.

Chemical peels work by creating a controlled
first- or second-degree burn of the skin. As the burn
heals, the body makes new collagen and elastin,
which gives the skin a more youthful appearance. A
chemical peel can resurface skin to reduce wrinkles

and fine lines around the eyes and mouth, sun spots, age spots, freckles, blotchy skin, mild scarring, some types of acne, and actinic keratoses or precancerous lesions.

Fresh-faced radiance past the age of 35 requires some assistance from specialist sources. I view peels as a continuum. I select the best chemical or chemical mix for each individual patient to tailor the treatment specifically to the patient's skin type and condition. A solution is applied using a sponge, cotton pad, cotton swab, or brush to the areas to be treated. The deeper a peel penetrates, the more visible results you can achieve, but the recovery period may be lengthier. Most peels can be performed on the face, neck, chest, hands, arms, and legs.

A peel treatment begins with cleansing the skin and removing all traces of grease with rubbing alcohol or acetone. The face is then rinsed with water and blown dry with a small fan. The peeling agent is applied so that all areas of the skin are covered evenly. It is usually started on the forehead at the hairline, then proceeds down one side of the face and down across the chin. This is repeated on the opposite side. The lower forehead is approached next, down the nose, across each cheek and finished with the upper lip. A grayish white film referred to as "frost" develops on the skin by the end of the application. The peeling solution is left in place for a few minutes and then thoroughly neutralized or removed with water. Excessive sunlight should be avoided for at least one week following a peel and one week prior to their next peel visit. In addition, a sunscreen with a minimum of SPF 15 should be applied as often as needed.

Types of Chemical Peels

Superficial peels. The most commonly performed chemical peels are superficial. These peels use mild chemical solutions like beta hydroxyl acid, glycolic acid, lactic acid, or salicylic acid, that lightly peel the skin with almost no recovery involved. They are typically done in a series to maintain results over time. Alpha hydroxy acid (AHA) peels performed in a physician's office require no anesthesia and the process usually takes 10 to 20 minutes. Your face may be slightly red and you can expect the redness to be followed by temporary flaking, dryness, and scaling until your skin adjusts to the treatments. Superficial peels are usually combined with a home skin care regimen for best results. The solution used will typically be adjusted for each treatment session based on your skin's response.

Medium peels. Jessner's solution, trichloroacetic acid (TCA) or other solutions are used to correct pigment problems, superficial blemishes, moderate sun damage, fine lines, and weathered skin. TCA peels are performed in a doctor's office.

Intravenous sedation is usually unnecessary because the chemical solution actually numbs the skin and cooling with ice or a fan after application is helpful. You may feel a warm or burning sensation which is followed by stinging. Your doctor will control the depth to which the chemical penetrates. TCA peels at strengths of 20% to 35% are usually performed on the full face to allow for maximum blending, but can also be used in regions such as under the eyelids and the upper lip in fair complexions. Medium-depth peels can take four to seven days to heal.

Deep peels. Deeper peel treatments such as phenol and croton oil peels are usually considered a one-time procedure. They produce more dramatic, long-term results on wrinkles, brown age spots, mild scarring, and precancerous growths. Because phenol peels result in permanently lightened skin, they are not recommended for darker skin tones. Phenol peels are usually performed in a surgicenter or hospital. A full-face deep peel requires intravenous sedation and cardiac monitoring, and generally takes one or two hours. Deeper peels can also be used on smaller areas of the face, such as the upper lip, at the time of a face-lift or other facial surgical procedure. Occlusive dressings are sometimes worn afterwards and the healing time is substantial. These peels are more akin to laser resurfacing and require that sunscreen be used at all times afterwards. Deep peels are not used on the neck or other parts of the body.

The deeper the peel, the better the result, the worse you look afterwards, and the longer it takes to heal. The lighter the peel, the more treatments you will need. Deeper peels have more of a risk of permanent skin bleaching (hypopigmentation), skin discoloration (hyperpigmentation), a line of demarcation, or scarring.

A Role for Microdermabrasion

Considered a light peel alternative, microdermabrasion entails blasting the face with sterile microparticles to rub off the very top skin layer, then vacuuming off the particles and the dead skin. Through a wandlike hand piece, tiny aluminum oxide or salt crystals are delivered at high velocity onto the skin surface and immediately vacuumed away with the same instrument, taking the top-most layer of dead skin cells with it. It exfoliates and gently resurfaces the skin, promoting the formation of new smoother skin. Microdermabrasion is usually performed on the face and neck, but can be performed on any part of the body including the hands, chest, arms, and legs.

Microdermabrasion can improve rough skin texture, some types of mild scarring, uneven pigmentation, and superficial brown spots. It is also useful for acne lesions, blackheads, some stretch marks, and fine wrinkles. One of its main advantages is that it can be safely used for all skin types. Each treatment will take approximately 30 minutes. A typical regimen consists of a series of four to eight treatments done at intervals of two to four weeks. Immediately after the procedure, makeup can be applied. The skin will have a pink glow that will fade within a few hours.

Microdermabrasion can improve the texture of the skin and can be combined with other resurfacing procedures such as peels and laser resurfacing. We typically use microdermabrasion on the stratum corneum, which results in signaling the lower layers of the epidermis to produce new skin cells and in stimulating the dermis to increase production of elastin and collagen. This process can quicken epidermal turnover and enhance youthful looks and the vitality of the skin.

Microdermabrasion is most beneficial for conditions such as hyperpigmentation and mild acne scarring, as well as skin texture problems. It is a versatile procedure that can be combined with techniques for more aggressive treatments.

Do-It-Yourself Peels:
Do They Get the Job Done?

When you can't get into your doctor's office for a professional peeling treatment, the next best thing is a home peel. There are many variations on the market that can be helpful to slough off surface debris and keep skin looking fresh and radiant. Home peels cannot go deep enough to smooth out lines and wrinkles or remove brown discoloration, but light peels are better than none at all.

You have to be careful not to overdo it if you are using at home peel systems, especially if you have dry or sensitive skin. The normal acid mantle of the skin has a pH that ranges between 4.0 and 5.5. Excessive use of acidic peeling agents can disrupt the acid mantle of healthy skin. Any elevation of the overall pH interferes with the skin's natural protective barrier and can result in dehydration, roughness, irritation, and flaking. If that occurs, the skin needs to be rehydrated with a mild rejuvenating moisturizer that can neutralize the alkaline ratio and reestablish a healthy ceramide barrier.

For oily or acne-prone skin, overly aggressive techniques or extremely alkaline products may end up stripping the skin of vital protective surface oils that can leave the skin red, irritated and inflamed, and vulnerable.

If you are using a home peel kit, avoid using additional glycolic acid products like cleansers and toners. You may find that you only need to do a light peel once a week or once every two weeks. The more oily or tough your skin is, the more frequently you may be able to use these products.

Skin-Saving Lasers and Light Sources

Due to widespread media coverage, lasers are now thought of as the best way for surgeons to cut tissue during surgery. Unfortunately, this is a misconception. For most operations, traditional cutting methods provide more precise control for the surgeon and smaller scars.

However, lasers do play an important role in skin resurfacing. Specifically, carbon dioxide (CO_2) lasers pulsed at very high frequencies are now being used by my practice and by other plastic surgeons instead of dermabrasion. By using a CO_2 laser, fine wrinkles around the mouth and eyelids can be markedly reduced with much less tissue destruction than seen with dermabrasion.

Lasers can also be used to treat acne scarring, acne lesions, age spots, birthmarks, and for hair removal. In addition, lasers are effective in the treatment of hemangiomas, red birthmarks, hyperpigmentation, moles, port wine stains, psoriasis, raised scars, repigmentation, skin cancers, thread veins, sun damage, varicose veins, and for tattoo removal. They can also be used to repigment skin that has been whitened or to treat scars that appear lighter than your normal skin color.

The CO_2 laser was one of the first lasers used by plastic surgeons and it became widely used by the early to mid-1990s. This technology offered dramatic results on aging skin, deep wrinkles, and acne scarring. However, laser resurfacing patients routinely had redness and crusting for weeks and their skin remained pink for up to three months in extreme cases. Over the years, we have learned more about

CO_2 laser technology and now can offer improved treatments with fewer side effects.

Unlike deeper lasers, nonablative lasers do not produce a deep burn, offering a much less invasive treatment that improves skin texture and tone by stimulating new collagen which serves to smooth out the skin. These treatments do not destroy the skin's outer tissue as they work their way down to stimulate collagen growth in the dermis. Nonablative lasers deliver controlled energy to the skin in slightly different ways, but the process is gradual and the softening of wrinkles occurs over time as the rejuvenated skin fibers reach the skin surface.

High-intensity light technology is now being used for skin contraction to tighten the skin for a nonsurgical lifting effect. Because of its collagen-stimulating capabilities, this technology is also being used to reduce wrinkles and fill in lines.

Lasers for Deep Resurfacing

Carbon dioxide (CO_2). The carbon dioxide (CO_2) laser is considered to be the workhorse of laser devices because of its ability to cause skin shrinkage and due to its dramatic results on deeper wrinkles. The CO_2 laser can reach deeper wrinkles because it heats tissue more intensely. As a result, it is a more invasive treatment with a longer recovery period.

When energy is delivered into the skin over a certain temperature, superficial tissues are vaporized and ablated, or destroyed. Typically, after a CO_2 laser treatment you will be required to apply an occlusive ointment for at least a week as the epidermis regenerates. One or two passes of the laser are more commonly used today to limit the amount of recovery time after the procedure.

Erbium:YAG. Erbium:YAG (yttrium aluminate garnet) laser technology has gained acceptance as the second cousin to the CO_2 laser, but without some of the side effects of a CO_2 device. The milder erbium:YAG laser works well on fine lines and wrinkles, mild sun damage, and scars. These lasers target the skin itself and the wavelengths are absorbed by water. Since most of our cells are predominantly water, these wavelengths are absorbed by the first cells they touch. The heat effects of the laser are scattered so that thin layers of tissue can be removed with precision while minimizing damage to surrounding skin.

An erbium:YAG laser treatment is like getting a medium-depth peel and works best for mild to moderate skin damage. If needed, treatment can be repeated in the future. I have also found that using nonablative photorejuvenation lasers after deeper resurfacing can also maintain results without the need for additional deeper procedures.

Nonablative Lasers and High-Intensity Light Sources

Lunchtime treatments with no downtime or redness are what people want today. Lasers and high-intensity light sources can accomplish this goal. In my experience, patients are willing to accept that the results will not be as dramatic, and that they will have to repeat these procedures more frequently. Many people simply do not want to go through a delayed healing process.

Nonablative lasers and high-intensity light sources work on the deeper layers of the skin without removing the top layer. They stimulate new collagen to smooth out the skin from deeper layers. These treatments do not produce a burn or destroy outer tissue as they work their way down to stimulate collagen growth in the dermis. Each device delivers controlled energy to the skin in slightly different ways. The process is gradual and the softening of wrinkles occurs over time as the rejuvenated skin fibers reach the skin surface. All of these systems require that treatments be repeated every four to six weeks and a minimum of three or four treatments are needed. The most common technologies are infrared lasers, visible light lasers, and broadband light sources.

Since lasers have a very long wavelength, they are relatively safe for a variety of skin types. There may be some discomfort, similar to a rubber band snapping against the skin. Topical anesthetic may be used to numb the skin for more superficial procedures. These systems are ideal for maintenance therapy after more aggressive or deeper resurfacing, or as part of a maintenance program in combination with skin care, peels, or microdermabrasion treatments. Most people see some improvement within 30 days and may continue to see improvements for up to 90 days. The newly formed collagen will then age at a normal rate and the procedure may be repeated as needed.

Intense pulsed light (IPL) sources. These multipurpose systems work by creating a wound in the small blood vessels within the dermis. This injury causes collagen and blood vessels under the top layer to contract. Light energy is delivered through the skin to remove redness and pigment, reduce pore size, to minimize fine lines, and to remove hair. After a few treatments, your skin will have a smoother, more even tone. If you have rosacea and facial flushing, you can expect to see a reduction in redness after each treatment. IPLs work for fine lines, particularly around the eyes and mouth, acne scars, brown spots, small veins, large pores, and chronic facial redness. They can also be used to treat areas on the neck, arms, chest, and hands.

Radio frequency waves. Devices utilizing radio frequency waves are being used to tighten loose skin on the face and body. They work by delivering deep, intense heat into the skin without injury to the epidermis. The system is comprised of a radio frequency (RF) generator, a controlled modular cooling system that houses a cryogen canister and related cooling control components, and a hand-held treatment tip that couples both the cryogen cooling and the RF heating device allowing for combined delivery of RF waves and cooling therapy. One or more treatments may be needed, and some anesthetic is necessary.

Light-emitting diode (LED) technology. Unlike laser technology that relies on high-powered coherent light to create heat energy, light-emitting diode (LED) photomodulation triggers the body to convert light energy into cell energy without damaging the tissues with heat. Treatment involves sitting in front of a panel of low-level LEDs. There is some evidence that this technology can turn off collagenase function, the enzyme that breaks down collagen, allowing collagen to last longer in the skin.

Repigmenting lasers. Excimer lasers are now being used to treat stretch marks, acne scars, burns, resurfaced skin, and depigmented skin. These light-based therapies improve the appearance of lighter scars by restoring pigment. Multiple treatments may be needed, and repigmentation can last up to several years depending on the extent of the hypopigmentation and the skin type being treated.

One of the most useful applications for these lasers is on face-lift scars that have spread or become white over time. Some women complain that they cannot wear their hair up after a face-lift, because the surgeon has placed the incision at the base of the hairline behind the ear, a location that can be very visible. In these cases, repigmenting lasers are sometimes used to repigment the incision scars so that they blend into the surrounding skin and become less noticeable.

Are You Ready For a Face-Lift?

5

"The general technique of a plastic operation differs slightly from that used in general surgery, in that the question of the ultimate appearance of the area of operation occupies a much more important place."

— Sir Harold D. Gilles
Plastic Surgery of the Face
(Oxford University Press, 1920)

The face continually changes as we age. However, cosmetic surgery ensures that you'll look younger than your chronological age. You will always look better after having a face-lift — regardless of when you do it.

Cosmetic surgery of the face now involves far more than just the "garden variety" face-lift. Remember, though, that face-lift surgery does not address the quality of your skin, blotches, age spots, or skin texture. Even if you have your heart set on a face-lift, continued maintenance of your skin, dermis, and musculature can improve skin quality, help a face-lift last longer, and postpone the need for your next lift.

Evaluating Your Face

As a person ages, skin cells divide more slowly, and the inner skin, or dermis, starts to thin. Fat cells beneath the dermis begin to atrophy, and the skin loses its elasticity as the underlying network of elastin and collagen fibers, which provides scaffolding for the surface layers, loosens and unravels. When pressed, the skin no longer springs back to its initial position; instead, it sags and forms furrows. The skin's ability to retain moisture diminishes and the sweat- and oil-secreting glands atrophy, depriving the skin of their protective water-lipid emulsions. As a consequence, the skin becomes dry and scaly. The ability of the skin to repair itself diminishes with age, so wounds are slower to heal. Frown lines between the eyebrows and crow's feet develop because of permanent small muscle contractions. Habitual facial expressions form characteristic lines, and gravity, exacerbating the situation, contributes to the formation of jowls and drooping eyelids. Eyebrows sometimes move up with age, due to continuous muscle strain to keep sagging brows elevated.

Aging is not limited to the surface of the skin. Time and photodamage take their toll on each layer of the skin and supportive tissues.

The Four Categories of Aging

1. Thickening of epidermal layer combined with diminished oil production creates a dull, lifeless and discolored appearance with small, fine wrinkle lines.

2. Thinning of the dermal layer with crumbling collagen and elastic fibers leads to further wrinkle formation, sagging, crepe-like texture, increased bruising and overall skin fragility.

3. Fat atrophy of the face leads to a sunken, tired appearance. As skin becomes less elastic, it also becomes drier. Underlying fat padding begins to disappear. With loss of underlying support by fat padding and connective tissues, the skin begins to sag and look less supple.

4. Thickening of the muscles of expression creates deeply grooved lines.

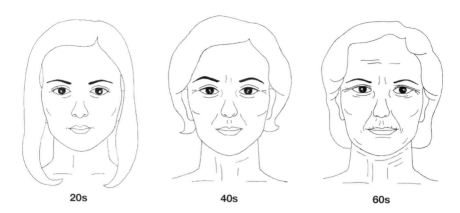

| 20s | 40s | 60s |

Facial Aging Changes

As in the rest of the body, the appearance of the face and neck changes with age. Muscle tone is lost, causing a flabby or droopy appearance. The jowls may begin to sag, contributing to a double chin. The nose lengthens slightly and may look more prominent. There is an increase in the number, size, and color of pigmented spots on the face.

The eyebrows and eyelashes lose pigment and turn gray. The skin around the eyelids becomes loose and wrinkled, resulting in crow's feet. The eye socket loses some of its fat pads, making the eyes look sunken. Drooping upper eyelids are fairly common and occasionally contribute to limitations in vision. The cornea may develop a grayish-white ring. The fat pad that lies below the eye starts to thin over time, creating a sunken look to the area, and the lower eyelid tends to droop, creating a "tear trough." The light that hits this area gives the illusion of a dark circle. Even the iris loses pigment, making most very elderly people appear to have gray or light blue eyes.

The bones begin to deteriorate slightly, most significantly in the inner ear which can cause changes in balance and hearing. Cartilage growth causes the ears to lengthen slightly. The ear canal becomes increasingly itchy and dry. Men may find that the ear hairs become longer, coarser, and more noticeable.

Loss of teeth can make the lips look thinner. The jawbone loses bone material, decreasing the size of the lower face, and often causing the forehead, nose and mouth to look more pronounced. Gums also recede, contributing to dental problems and changes in appearance of the mouth. The thyroid gland can look more pronounced on the front of the neck. Noses tend to enlarge and droop, as nasal cartilage continues to grow throughout life.

Dr. Cohen's Formula for Tracking Age Changes

Aging doesn't happen overnight and everyone's face ages differently. Some people find themselves with greater jowling earlier than others, while some have increased laxity of the neck or wrinkling on the cheeks. Adults age in spurts just as children grow in spurts, and these aging spurts are often associated with stressful periods in life. We tend to grow accustomed to seeing ourselves in a mirror every day and mentally block out imperfections. You don't just wake up one morning and wonder how all these changes occurred. Although they have been there all the time, you may not have noticed age-related changes — until you see a recent photo. A photo is a reverse image of ourselves and allows us to see our

Fade Out

- Skin pales
- Hair color dulls
- Eyebrows lighten
- Lips lose pigment
- Eyelashes diminish

Skin Changes

- Redness and broken capillaries appear
- Wrinkles form along expression lines
- Surface becomes rough and dull
- Brown spots and pigmentation appear
- Skin dries out
- Pores enlarge
- Circles around eyes darken

Sagging

- Eyebrows droop to below the bony rim
- Eyes close in, appear crowded
- Eyes look smaller
- Tip of nose drops and cartilage enlarges
- Cheeks move forward
- Neck sags
- Corners of mouth turn down
- Fat accumulates under eyes and along jaw line

flaws as they truly are. Think about how many people you know who don't believe they photograph well.

One tool I use in my communication with patients is a computer-based imaging system that allows us to take a photo and then modify the image on the computer screen. By doing this, we can show a patient an image of a reasonable outcome of a cosmetic procedure. This also gives patients the opportunity to show the doctor what they like or dislike about their current features or a proposed outcome.

This state-of-the-art computer imaging technology helps to alleviate unrealistic self-images that patients may harbor. We can demonstrate what can and cannot be done surgically, and judge whether these improvements are going to make the patient happy. Most importantly, computer imaging involves you, the patient, in planning the surgery. This aspect is frequently missing from many preoperative consultations. After all, it is *your* face in question and only you should decide what should be improved or changed.

The Eyes and Brows

Eyelid skin, because of its composition and lack of oil glands, is more prone to wrinkling. The eyelids age in several ways. Sun exposure will weaken the elastic fibers that keep eyelid skin taut. Droopy eyelids or puffy lower eyelids often run in families, and are as common in men as they are in women. Protruding fatty tissue from the eye sockets that causes bags can be an inherited trait that shows up early in life, or it can be the result of aging.

At first, bags or sagging may be most noticeable when you are tired, then they become visible all of the time. Eyelid skin thins, stretches, and loosens as it ages, and eye muscles weaken. Fat that cushions the eyeball moves forward around the eyes. Puffiness results when the fat pad that cushions the eye begins to pull away from the bony eye socket and sags. Gravity has its effects on the eyes as well. As the upper eyelids become heavier and fuller with age, they may sag resulting in "hooding" over the eyes.

Eyelid surgery, referred to as blepharoplasty, should never compromise the functional elements of the eyelids for the sake of aesthetics. In blepharoplasty, excess fat, skin, and if needed, muscle are removed from the upper and/or lower eyelids. Blepharoplasty can reduce droopy or hooded eyelids, restore the contour to the lids and eliminate the protruding fat bags under the eyes. In some cases, eyelid surgery may also correct ptosis, which is severe hooding of the upper eyelids that can obstruct peripheral vision and reduce the range of upward vision.

The typical healing period after eyelid surgery is brief. Many patients are swollen for a period of seven to 10 days. Some bruising, progressing to mild discoloration of the cheek surface, is often seen for up to two weeks after surgery. The major risk associated with eyelid surgery is ectropion, which is defined as a pull-down of the eyelids due either to excess skin removal or the formation of scar tissue. In most cases, ectropion is transient in nature. If it occurs, it typically responds well to daily massage or taping of the eyelids while the

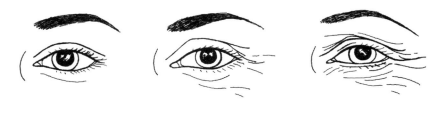

Aging Eye Changes

patient is sleeping. If you have a history of dry-eye syndrome, low tear production, hyperthyroidism, or very prominent eyes, you may not be considered a good candidate for cosmetic eyelid surgery.

In some patients, excess fat and skin in the upper eyelid alone cause drooping of the lids and brow. In others, drooping of the brow itself causes the appearance of excess skin and fullness. Some patients who request upper eyelid surgery are better candidates for brow-lifts, which can now be done endoscopically. Some patients require both an eyelid and brow-lift procedure to optimize the outcome. Only a thorough physical examination will allow for an adequate diagnosis of the underlying problem.

There are two basic techniques for brow-lifting: the more traditional coronal brow-lift, and variations of an endoscopic forehead lift. For a coronal brow-lift, an incision is made slightly behind the natural hairline, running from ear to ear across the top of the head, where a headset would sit. The incision is usually made well behind the hairline so that the scar is not visible. If your hairline is high or receding, the incision may be placed just at the hairline, so as not to move the forehead back.

Another method, called the midbrow-lift, involves placing the incisions in the deep horizontal forehead furrows. This technique is usually reserved for men. In most cases, the scar heals very well and can be imperceptible. In Asia, placing the incisions to raise the brows at the eyebrow just above the hair follicles is a popular technique that often works nicely.

One of the most exciting advances in cosmetic surgery recently has been the use of the endoscope in facial rejuvenation procedures. An endoscope is a small camera which can be inserted through a tiny incision in the skin and which transmits an image of the underlying tissues to a video screen. Endoscopy has been applied by orthopedic surgeons to treat cartilage damage in joints (arthroscopy) and by gynecologists to examine pelvic organs (laparoscopy). Plastic surgeons now perform brow-lifts through several tiny incisions in the scalp. Until recently, the only way a brow-lift could be performed was with an "ear to ear" incision.

There have been many advancements in the methods of fixation of the brow in endoscopic brow-lifting, resulting in new and improved techniques to hold the tissues in place. Secure fixation offers long-term, predictable results from an endoscopic brow-lift procedure. I have used various fixation techniques and currently prefer to use an implant called an Endotine instead of sutures or metallic screws. Unlike earlier methods, this device does not need to be removed and puts less stress on the hair follicles.

In some cases, we can even perform full face-lifts via the endoscope. In those patients whose

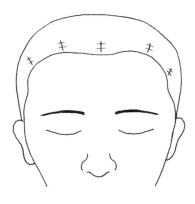

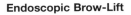

Endoscopic Brow-Lift

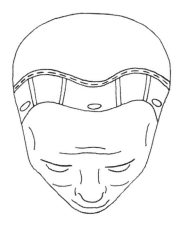

Open Brow-Lift

complaints are of midface and jowl sagging rather than excess skin, a face-lift can be performed through several small puncture wounds in the scalp and a lower eyelid incision. The best candidates for this procedure are those patients in their 30s and 40s with good skin tone. These minimal incisions for face-lift surgery have allowed the treatment of the aging face to extend to much younger patients with significantly improved results.

New Techniques in Face- and Neck-Lifts

A well-done face-lift will not change your looks or make you look like a different person; that is not the goal. Instead, it is a restoration of the natural facial contours, particularly of the neck and jowl area. Tissues are elevated to where they started out and the underlying musculature is tightened, leaving the patient with a refreshed, harmonious appearance. When you spot someone who has undergone a face-lift who looks radically different, it is usually a sign that more than just a face-lift has been performed. For example, facial implants or nose reshaping will make you appear slightly different than if a "stand alone" face-lift is done.

A common mistake many women make when considering a facial rejuvenation procedure is thinking that their face stops at their chin line. Neck skin is thin and gravity tends to attack the neck early. There are fewer oil glands in the neck, so it craves hydration. (I recommend using an antiaging cream for the neck area nightly. My number one choice for the neck is retinoic acid, complemented by regular sunscreen use.)

However, when your neck is truly sagging,

creams can no longer get the job done and the only effective remedy is surgery. Slack skin and muscles need to be redraped, lifted, and tightened to restore a smooth swan-like appearance to the neck.

The face and neck are common areas that show the effects of gravity, sun damage, and the stresses of daily life. Areas of the face that are improved with face and neck lift surgery are the jowls, wrinkles of the cheek, and laxity of the neck, commonly exemplified by the "turkey gobbler" neck. Indeed, the best candidates for a face-lift are either a man or a woman whose face and neck have begun to sag, but whose skin still has remaining elasticity. (The areas most difficult to improve with face-lift surgery are the nasolabial folds, or the crease where the cheek meets the area of the lips.)

On average, women considering face-lifts today are in their mid-40s, and men are around 50. Women of color may not need a face-lift until their mid-50s, due to their increased skin thickness and the fact that they are less prone to premature wrinkling.

Perhaps this relatively early age for face-lifts can also be attributed to the desire not to look 20 years younger, but to look rejuvenated before your friends and family are aware that you have had surgical intervention. Face-lift surgery has become more common among a younger patient population and more accepted as a rite of passage, rather than a frivolous self-indulgence. The ideal time for a face-lift is when you think you need it, and this varies in every case. While face-lifts can be done successfully in patients in their 70s or 80s, at that stage there is usually more to be done and results will not be as good or last as long.

On average, women considering face-lifts today are in their mid-40s, and men are around 50.

In my experience, male patients usually want just a neck procedure done instead of a full face-lift. Their chief complaints are loose skin of the neck and jowling. In some cases, a neck lift can be accomplished in men by using a "z-plasty" incision to redrape the excess skin of the neck and tighten the muscles. This involves placing a z-shaped scar along the anterior or front of the neck, which usually heals well after surgery.

Preconditioning the Skin for Surgery

Good skin care is an important element of our practice. It allows our patients to get back to work and get on with their lives. A comprehensive skin care regimen is critical to a good surgical outcome. If you have a face-lift with all the trimmings but have old-looking, dry, and dehydrated skin with brown spots and old scars, your face-lift may not look as good as it should. We recommend that all our face-lift, brow-lift, and eyelid surgery patients start a good skin care regimen three to six weeks prior to surgery. This serves the dual purpose of making the skin healthier, while aiding the healing in order to enhance the results of surgery.

Face-Lift Fundamentals

The risks and complications associated with face-lift surgery include hematoma (collection of blood underneath the skin that must be surgically drained), infection, prolonged numbness, and poor scarring. Injury to the nerves of the facial muscles can be seen in one out of several thousand patients. Fortunately, this condition is usually temporary due to the extensive crossover seen in facial nerve anatomy. Injury to the nerve related to feeling in the ear can also be seen; however, this is is also infrequent. Infections of the skin can occur, but are more common in patients who smoke. Mild asymmetries after surgery are noted in some patients, but these will usually pass with time, or are easily corrected with minor touch-up procedures.

The type of anesthesia used during face-lift surgery varies from local anesthesia with intravenous sedation to complete general anesthetic. When a face-lift is combined with other longer procedures, such as a brow-lift and upper and lower eyelid surgery, general anesthesia is often chosen. Face-lifts can be performed in an office-based operating room or in an outpatient surgery center or hospital. When face-lifts are performed as a solo procedure, hospitalization is usually not required. The surgery can take two to three hours and longer if more procedures are being performed at the same time. It is common to combine face-lift surgery with other aspects of facial rejuvenation, such as upper and lower eyelid blepharoplasty, brow-lift, lip-lift, laser resurfacing, and fat injections. Staged procedures are sometimes recommended due to the increased propensity for scarring when face-lifts, for example, are combined with full face laser resurfacing.

The incisions for face-lift surgery usually begin above the hairline at the temples and extend in front of the ear or just inside the ear cartilage. The incisions then continue behind the earlobe and on into the scalp or hairline. The surgeon then separates the skin from the underlying fat and muscle from below. Excess fat, such as in the area of jowls and neck, is removed

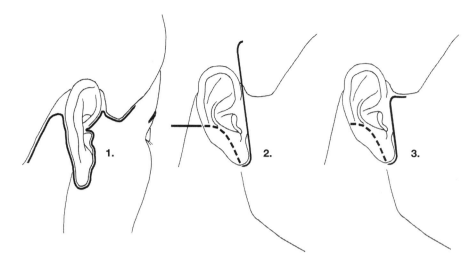

1. Standard Face-Lift
2. Modified Face-Lift
3. S-Lift or Mini Face-Lift

either by direct excision or by liposuction. I will also tighten the underlying muscles of the face to give the face-lift more longevity.

Face-lift procedures are constantly changing and the concept of facial rejuvenation has evolved to encompass a total approach to remodeling, not just pulling the skin taut. No single formula is right for everyone; the surgical plan should be customized for each individual patient. Modified techniques may reduce a portion of the scar by eliminating the scar that extends behind the ear. A modified face-lift (also referred to as a "minimal" or "mini" face-lift, or in some circles as an "S-lift") is a good option for younger patients who do not require as much correction. It is less invasive, which translates to reduced swelling, scarring, bruising, and risk, and can be done under local anesthesia alone.

Postoperatively, there is minimal discomfort associated with all facial rejuvenation surgery, and it is easily relieved by pain medication. Some surgeons choose to use a drainage tube inserted through a separate incision, which is removed one or two days after surgery. Bandages, if needed, are usually removed soon after surgery.

Most patients are able to go out in public in approximately 10 to 14 days. Strenuous activities should be avoided for at least two weeks after surgery. This is to help prevent collection of blood underneath the areas of surgery. Camouflage make-up can be worn soon after surgery to allow the patient to appear in public. (A green base balances red hues and a purple or mauve base balances bruising.) In the immediate postoperative period, the features appear rather distorted due to swelling and bruising. It takes two to three months for all facial swelling to dissipate after face-lift surgery.

As their new, more youthful face emerges from the underlying bruising, most patients are delighted with the outcome. While having a face-lift turns back the clock, it does not stop it. Revision is frequently necessary in five or 10 years to continue the lasting effects of the facial rejuvenation surgery.

The Matter of Hair Loss

Hair loss is one of the most common fears of face-lift patients and can sometimes result from a face-lift or brow-lift. It is usually a temporary condition and regrowth occurs within the first three to four months after face-lift surgery.

Hair loss is common in women as well as men, and can be even more devastating for a woman since it often comes as a shock. Unlike men who tend to lose hair in one concentrated area, women are prone to a thinning that starts at the top and gradually spreads. If the cause is largely genetic, the use of topical minoxidil is a good place to start. More serious hair loss conditions require micro- and minigraft transplantation. For women who are already experiencing thinning hair and contemplating a lift, I prescribe a course of minoxidil before and/or after surgery used twice daily every day for a period of four months. For male patients, I usually prescribe Propecia®, since it is often more effective. Additionally, women may benefit from spironolactone, which is a mild diuretic and male hormone blocker.

Enhancing Your Bone Structure

Facial shaping by removing, repositioning or adding soft tissue, rather than by tightening the skin and muscles alone, is considered the key to achieving optimal results in facial rejuvenation. Facial implant surgery may be performed to build up various facial features to give the face a more balanced and less flattened appearance. Implants are placed under the skin to build up contours, and areas of over-prominent tissues may be reduced to minimize contour imbalances. Typical regions of contour change include the cheekbones, the jawbone and chin, as well as the lips in some cases.

To augment a facial contour, material is implanted deeply below the skin surface and secured with permanent stitches into surrounding tissues, so it cannot move. There is a wide variety of implant materials, shapes and sizes on the market including silicone, Gore-Tex, Medpor®, elastomer and human tissues (see Chapter 4). Facial implants are typically fashioned from solid and semisolid materials, as opposed to the gel- or saline-filled implants that are used in breast augmentation.

Rejuvenating the Ears

Ear surgery, or otoplasty, is usually performed to set prominent ears back closer to the head or to reduce the size of one or both ears if they are too large in proportion to the size and shape of the face. Although the operation is most commonly performed on children (ideally at age seven to eight), it can also be performed on adults. Besides protruding ears, there are a variety of other ear conditions that can be improved. Surgery can also be undertaken to improve large or stretched earlobes, or lobes that have large creases due to aging or years of wearing heavy earrings. It is common to have an earlobe repair or earlobe reduction done in conjunction with face-lift surgery. When only one ear appears to protrude, surgery is usually performed on both ears to create a good balance. Even after undergoing an otoplasty, there is no guarantee that your ears will be perfectly symmetrical.

Nasal Refinements

Nasal surgery is perhaps the most demanding cosmetic surgery, since it deals with both form and function and requires considerable skill. Ethnic variations in nasal anatomy also make the operation more technically and aesthetically difficult to master for the surgeon. Indeed, rhinoplasty can be used to alter ethnic characteristics, or to improve on features within the framework of a patient's ethnicity.

The concept of nasal refinement has changed dramatically over the past few decades. Originally, the operation was typically undertaken to reduce the size and projection of the nose. The days of "scooped" noses have given way to an era of more subtle and balanced rhinoplasty, using techniques that give the cosmetic surgeon many more options for reshaping the nose.

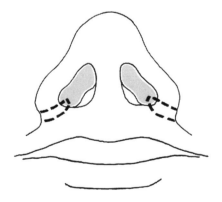

Alar Base Resection to Narrow Nostrils

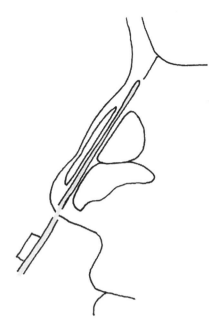

Reshaping the Nasal Dorsum

Because the nose is the focal point of the face, its cosmetic alteration can have a profound impact on one's appearance. A large bump, a broad tip or a wide nasal pyramid can lead to facial imbalances that may draw attention away from more attractive features such as beautiful eyes or full lips. In many cases, augmentation — adding either cartilage or synthetic materials to raise certain areas of the nose — has replaced traditional complete reduction rhinoplasties.

Most nasal surgeries are performed through incisions inside the nose. The exception to this is an "open rhinoplasty," a technique using small incisions made at the columella (the island of skin separating the nostrils). Very wide-based noses will sometimes require external incisions to narrow flaring nostrils. However, the preponderance of nose reduction surgery can be carried out through inconspicuous incisions inside the nose.

In general, the nose can be broken down into several major areas which will benefit from correction. The tip is defined as the area just above the nostrils. It is the area of the nose that projects the furthest from the face. In some people, this projection is inadequate, while in others it is too great. Either of these anatomic variations can be corrected through surgery. A broad or boxy tip can be refined and an inadequate tip can be augmented.

The middle third of the nose is often characterized by a substantial bump. This bump is composed of cartilage and is reduced simply by removing extra cartilage through incisions made inside the nose.

The upper portion of the nose is made up of the nasal bones. Nasal bone structure will contribute to a large or wide nose. This can be reduced by rasping or by nasal fractures. Finally, the width of the nose can be addressed by small incisions inside the nose, which allow the nasal bones to be moved closer together.

In certain ethnic groups, augmentation of the nose is desirable. It is now possible to augment the nose either with a patient's own tissues or with safe, inert synthetic materials. This allows a cosmetic surgeon to either raise the profile or improve the nasal tip. Altering the angle at which the nose meets the face can also be accomplished with similar techniques.

Functional and cosmetic nasal surgeries are

often combined. Many people suffer from chronic, obstructed nasal breathing. This is usually due to either a deviated septum or to enlargement of the bones on the sides of the nose known as turbinates. Both of these problems are easily corrected and can be treated with or without altering the appearance of the nose.

Recovery from nasal surgery is remarkably swift. After a complete rhinoplasty, the average patient will have a splint on the outside of their nose for five to seven days. Most people are somewhat bruised from the surgery around the eyes for 10 to 14 days. Camouflage make-up can be used to diminish the bruising after the first several days. Functional nasal surgery often requires that internal splints be placed inside the nostrils. These cannot be seen and are removed approximately two to three weeks after the operation.

The amount of pain associated with nasal surgery is usually minimal. The nose will feel stuffy and stiff at first, and there may be some crusting. It is important to abstain from heavy lifting, bending or straining to avoid bleeding. Breathing is sometimes impaired in the immediate postoperative period, especially when functional nasal surgery is done. This improves as the swelling subsides over the ensuing weeks.

The final outcome of the operation is not seen for six months to one year since swelling persists for some time in the area of the nose. The last area in which the effects of nasal surgery can be seen is at the tip where swelling usually persists the longest.

Revision nasal surgery is required in 5-10% of all patients undergoing surgery of the nose. The reason for this is related to shifting and twisting of cartilage in the postoperative period and scar tissue formation at the area of the operation. Unfortunately, the need for revision cannot be predicted based on the preoperative examination. Twisting of cartilage and shifting of the nasal bones which were once straight is also common. There is a significant interplay among numerous structures in the nose that undergo alteration during the surgery. The revision rate is high because of the continued shifts and stresses in the postoperative period. The good news is that in most cases, revisions are quite minor.

Nasal surgery is performed on an outpatient basis either under general anesthesia, or local anesthesia with intravenous sedation. We prefer for patients to complete maturation of the facial skeleton prior to undertaking nasal surgery. In girls, this means no rhinoplasty before the age of 12 to 13, and in males, one would typically not proceed with rhinoplasty until the age of 15 to 16. The upper age range is driven by patient desire.

The nose continues to grow as we get older and age-related changes of the nose such as a drooping tip can be seen. A drooping nasal tip is frequently repaired along with other facial rejuvenation procedures. Nasal surgery is often combined with correction of other areas of facial imbalance, such as a weak or overly projected chin. These ancillary procedures should be recommended by a plastic surgeon when evaluating the face as a whole.

Personally, nasal surgery is one of my favorite procedures because it can dramatically change the patient's overall appearance and greatly improve self-confidence and self-esteem.

Presurgical Considerations, Healing and Recovery

As a plastic surgeon, I am completely engaged in the science of wound healing. In my practice, I devote considerable energy to accelerating the healing process for my patients. We put patients on a strict preoperative skin care program to insure a smooth recovery.

Fortunately, the trend in cosmetic surgery is toward less invasive techniques with fewer and smaller incisions, as well as faster-acting anesthetic agents with fewer side effects. Today, more than half of all cosmetic surgeries are done on an outpatient basis, either at a hospital, surgery center or in a doctor's operating room. Recovery usually takes place in your own home, so there is less disruption of your lifestyle and schedule.

It is normal to become anxious before undergoing surgery. Stress causes hormones to be released that, in turn, result in symptoms like headaches, high blood pressure, sleeplessness, and irritability. The emotional impact of surgery is coupled with the physical nature of the trauma to the body. For some patients, the fear of having anesthesia or losing control is worse than the anxieties regarding the surgery and its outcome combined.

Outpatient surgery is not right for everyone. If you have any medical condition like diabetes or hypertension, or you are over 65, you may require hospitalization overnight. Same-day surgery may not be ideal if you live alone, or if you don't want to bother family or friends to apply ice compresses or change your dressings. Mothers with small children without nannies, or anyone who lives more than a two-hour drive from the nearest hospital should think twice about outpatient surgery. Ambulatory procedures put a major burden on your caretaker, and it's a big favor to ask of a casual acquaintance or friend to care for you postoperatively. Home care nurses are available to provide care for a day or two as an alternative.

Generally, bruising resolves within the first three weeks following any cosmetic procedure. In some cases, there may be a slight discoloration or light bruising for a longer period if you have had excessive bleeding during surgery or postsurgical complications that may delay healing. The initial swelling will resolve within the first few weeks, but may be present for several months or longer. The use of tissue glue or fibrin sealant intraoperatively may cut down on the amount of bruising and swelling that results. In my practice, tumescent local anesthesia is also instrumental in minimizing bruising for facial rejuvenation procedures. Steroids given intravenously preoperatively and orally postoperatively are also used to help reduce swelling.

Some surgeons will also prescribe topical vitamin K cream or arnica gel after surgery to decrease bruising. (Oral vitamin K can potentially help but it is associated with blood clotting and is no longer used.) Arnica tablets taken before surgery may also be useful as a prophylactic.

We require our patients to give up caffeine, aspirin and aspirin-containing drugs, vitamin E, ibuprofen, and any other medications including vitamins and supplements that could thin the blood, disrupt the blood-clotting process or facilitate bruising. Aspirin, for example, is a potent anticoagulant that can cause excessive bleeding. Some supplements and herbal teas may also interfere with the effects of anesthesia and bleeding, and should be discontinued. In some cases, antibiotics will be prescribed prior to surgery, as in patients with a history of mitral valve prolapse, a heart murmur or previous hip or joint replacement.

If you have a history of bad scarring or thickened scars such as keloids, or delayed healing from past surgical procedures, we like to know about this ahead of time so that we can take precautions. In general, the immediate scars will remain somewhat thickened and red for weeks or months, then gradually become less obvious, eventually fading to thin white lines.

Smokers or nicotine patch users have increased risks in surgery because nicotine constricts the blood vessels, decreases blood flow to tissues and greatly increases the chance of scarring. In some cases, smokers can actually lose a portion of skin due to decreased oxygen flow into the skin and impaired blood flow. Nicotine substitutes and smoker's aids also increase the risk of poor healing, skin sloughing, scabbing and crusting. These risks are significantly reduced if you stop smoking at least two weeks before surgery and wait until you are completely healed before starting again. We prefer that you quit smoking entirely.

Inflammation is the normal reaction of tissue after any injury. The immediate response of the

Herbal supplements containing echinacea, ginseng, garlic, gingko biloba, St. John's wort, ephedra, and ma huang should be stopped for three weeks before and after surgery, along with aspirin, anti-inflammatories, and vitamin E, all of which can cause bleeding and increased bruising.

Good wound care will minimize the inflammatory response, speed healing, and minimize scarring.

blood supply to the area is a constriction of the vessels. This is followed immediately by vasodilation that allows fluid to exit the capillaries and flood the area. Chemicals in the plasma and on injured tissues attract white blood cells that enter the area and start to clean up foreign material, bacteria and dead cells. Accumulation of a large number of white blood cells leads to pus in the wound. Eventually the clot is replaced by granulation tissue, a connective tissue with a rich blood supply. Scars are red because of the ample blood supply, and the color gradually fades to white as the vascularization decreases and the collagen matrix matures. When the coverage of the wound surface beneath the scab is complete, the scab sloughs off and the epidermis begins to keratinize. Remodeling of the collagen matrix may continue for years depending on individual genetics and age.

I often tell my patients that how you heal is between you and God, and your choice of parents. However, there are some techniques that can be employed to refine surgery and improve the healing process. Deeper incisions require some sort of manual closure such as sutures, staples, or tapes. Sutures are made of foreign material like "cat gut," or synthetic polyglycolic acid derivatives, nylon, silk, or stainless steel. The first two examples are absorbable and the others must be removed. Using fine suture material with minimal tension on the wound can limit any additional tissue damage, inflammation, and scarring (which is where choosing your surgeon comes into play). Wounds in areas where there is less blood supply that heal slowly, or wounds in high-stress areas, require larger suture material and stitches that must remain in longer. Sutures may sometimes be removed after only a few days to minimize scarring, for example, in the delicate eyelid area.

Ultrasound and electrical stimulation are effective methods of increasing blood flow and treating surgical wounds. When ultrasound waves enter the body they are absorbed more readily by muscle, tendons, and bone than by fat. Postoperatively, our overriding goal is to reduce this swelling quickly to eliminate any further cellular damage. Low-intensity ultrasound can help advance the healing process in some cases. When there is substantial scar tissue or swelling, ultrasound therapy can be used to break up hardening and ease patient distress.

Any patient who is undergoing surgery should be cautious about the treatments they receive before and after the procedure. The timing of the procedure must be safe and appropriate, and beneficial to the surgical outcome. For example, cosmetic surgery patients may be hypersensitive after surgery and may not tolerate the pulling sensation created by the suction device of a microdermabrader for four to six weeks postoperatively. We typically take our patients off all acidic skin care compounds for a period of two to three weeks after surgery as the skin is healing and may be more prone to irritation. If laser resurfacing has been performed, you should follow your doctor's instruction to the letter, as the skin may be extremely reactive at that stage.

- Initiate the process with a microdermabrasion treatment or superficial glycolic peel once per week for three to four weeks to slough off epidermal build-up.

- Pretreat the skin with Retin-A at night, preferably with a 0.1% formulation if your skin can tolerate it. For more sensitive or delicate skin types, start with 0.025% or 0.05% cream instead.

- If laser resurfacing is being planned, skin may also be pretreated with a lightening agent like hydroquinone or Kligman's formula (hydroquinone and Retin-A compound).

- Daily use of SPF 20 plus topical vitamin C serum; avoid sun exposure.

- Take beta carotene, vitamin C, vitamin B complex daily for two weeks before and after surgery.

- Avoid drinking more than one to two glasses of wine for two weeks before surgery; alcohol is dehydrating.

- Stop smoking or nicotine substitutes or patches for two to three weeks before and after surgery.

- On the morning of surgery, do not use anything on your face including moisturizer or sunscreen.

The Role of Good Nutrition

Although overall balanced nutrition is the starting point for successful healing of surgical wounds, the most recent research has emphasized the role and intake of certain specific nutrients. If you are considering plastic surgery, or have already had a surgical procedure, you know that you should anticipate some swelling, bruising, and tenderness. The prevention of infection and the proper healing of the wound is of key concern. A vitamin deficiency can result in a slow healing process or even hinder your body from effectively fighting a potential infection. Therefore, it is important to maintain a well-balanced diet including a wide variety of fruits and vegetables.

Take a moment to critically assess your nutritional habits and try to fill the gaps. In addition, if your diet is deficient in certain nutrients, you should consider adding recommended nutritional supplements to your daily regime. A good multivitamin (containing only trace amounts of vitamin E which can cause bleeding), is necessary to help you fight disease and to keep your skin healthy.

Make sure you know what to expect after surgery so there are no surprises. Surgery is not a perfect science, but the more you know, the better your surgical outcome will be. Listen carefully to all risks and complications associated with the proposed surgery. It is not a day at the spa, and yes, complications can arise. Understand the time line involved in the healing process. Three months is 90 days for everyone! You should trust your surgeon and be confident that if a complication does arise, your surgeon will address it.

Heavenly Bodies

6

"Is not plastic surgery an art and the plastic surgeon an artist? The plastic surgeon works with living flesh as his clay, and his work of art is the attempted achievement of normalcy in appearance and function."

—Jerome Pierce Webster
Professor of Surgery, Columbia University
1888-1974

Whether your ultimate goal is to look great in your clothes, fit into a smaller size or look better in the nude, there are numerous surgical and nonsurgical options to consider that can enhance and rejuvenate your body and the skin that protects it.

Body Basics:
Veins, Age Spots, Stretch Marks and Other Imperfections

Flawless skin is a fleeting concept. Everyone has imperfections they would like to erase, and some tend to be more treatable than others. The skin of your extremities and your body can appear younger, unblemished, and healthier through various treatment options.

If you are having cosmetic surgery or less-invasive treatments to make your face look younger, don't forget your hands, arms, and chest. These areas, which are frequently exposed to the effects of the sun, may still reveal your age. The cumulative effects of aging, sun, and exposure to chemicals can result in brown spots, uneven pigmentation, skin cancers, thinning skin, and prominent veins. Brown spots and red lesions, for example, are now treated with lasers. Lasers can also be utilized to reduce age spots on hands, legs, the chest, and other locations, so that a newly lifted face can be complemented by youthful hands and neck.

Although we tend to think of skin aging primarily on the face, the body is also susceptible to the ravaging effects of time. Exfoliating and rejuvenating agents can be just as effective for treating the skin of the body. Microdermabrasion is a popular treatment for the body, as are superficial peels. They gently slough and polish the skin, reducing areas of discoloration and moderate sun damage. Intense pulsed light (IPL) systems are also used to reduce imperfections of the hands, legs and chest, and to stimulate the skin for a collagen-producing effect. The benefits of these treatments — especially for women entering menopause when estrogen levels drop and the skin dries out and thins — include improvement in skin texture and dermal thickening which combats the inevitable loss of firmness that comes with age.

Another common complaint is spider veins, those small, thin veins that lie close to the surface of the skin that appear as small clusters of red, blue or purple lines on the thighs, calves and ankles. Although you cannot prevent them, the simplest treatment methods are sclerotherapy and lasers. Many factors cause the development of spider veins, including heredity, pregnancy and other events that cause hormonal shifts, weight gain, activities that require prolonged sitting or standing, and wearing high heels.

The most common treatment calls for the veins to be injected with a sclerosing solution, which causes them to rupture and then fade. After each session, the veins should appear lighter. Usually, two or more sessions are required to achieve the best results. No vein treatment can prevent new veins from appearing in the future, and if you are prone to getting them, you can expect to see more turn up. The treated veins will be gone permanently, but the process may need to be repeated, depending upon the degree of severity and the number of veins to be treated.

Possible risks associated with spider vein removal include blood clots, inflammation, skin slough and wounds, allergic reaction to the solution, and pigmentation irregularities. Spider vein treatment is a relatively simple procedure that requires no anesthesia, so it can be performed in an outpatient setting, such as your doctor's office. Tight-fitting support hose are normally prescribed to guard against blood clots for 72 hours or longer. When the dressings are removed, you may notice bruising and reddish areas at the injection sites. If this occurs, the bruises will lessen and disappear within the first month. Some people experience a residual brownish pigmentation, which may take up to a year to completely fade.

Varicose veins differ from spider veins in that they tend to bulge and are larger and darker in color. They also are more likely to cause pain and involve more serious vein disorders. Sclerotherapy may sometimes be used to treat varicose veins but surgical treatment is usually necessary. You will be checked for signs of more serious "deep vein" problems, often indicated by swelling, soreness, or skin changes at the ankle. A hand-held Doppler ultrasound device is sometimes used to detect any backflow within the venous system. If other problems are identified, your plastic surgeon may refer you to a vascular surgeon for further evaluation.

For years, stretch marks held out little hope for a good solution. Advances in laser technology now offer effective treatments to reduce the pigment in stretch marks so that they fade away. Stretch marks occur in the dermis which makes them more difficult to treat than if they appeared on the surface of the skin. When the dermis is constantly stretched over time, the skin loses elasticity and the connective fibers break.

Depending on your natural skin coloring, stretch marks may start out as raised pink, reddish brown, or dark brown striations that turn a deeper violet or purple. Gradually, the marks flatten and fade to a color a few shades lighter than your natural skin tone and take on a translucent quality. They usually become less noticeable over time. Mature stretch marks do not respond as well to topical or laser therapies as newer, pigmented marks. Stretch marks can appear anywhere on the body where the skin has been stretched; for example, the breasts, thighs, and abdomen. They are more likely to appear in areas where fat is stored.

Laser treatments with IPL systems and nonablative lasers like the Cool Touch™, NLite™ and others brands will not entirely remove stretch marks. Their objective is to fade the pigment and flatten the stretch marks. These lasers target pigment in the skin, so faded, flesh-colored marks do not respond well. A series of treatments will be required for visible results, and laser therapy is often combined with microdermabrasion and topical remedies including retinoic acid and an alpha hydroxy acid (AHA) for best results.

The Dimple Effect:
An Anticellulite Attack Plan

Cellulite is caused by bands of fibrous tissue that connect the muscle to the skin. If these bands are tight, and the fat between the muscle and the skin is compressed, there will be a "cottage cheese" or "orange peel" look to the skin. Almost all women have cellulite, stemming primarily from genetic predisposition, hormonal changes, and weight gain. Over the years, various cellulite cures have come and gone, and none offered a treatment program that worked over the long term.

As a plastic surgeon, I know firsthand that liposuction does not reduce cellulite. However, breaking up the fibrous bands using a liposuction cannula with a sharp, V-pronged cutting edge may have the effect of severing the connective tissues that are at the root of dimpling. In my experience, using this technique offers little relief from chronic cellulite, which often worsens with age. The effects are largely temporary, and in many patients we have seen the dimples reappear. Mechanical roller massage therapy or endermologie has been used as a treatment for cellulite and as an adjunct to liposuction. Long-term results of this noninvasive therapy have not been established clinically or scientifically; however, many patients claim that they do see a difference after an intense course of treatments.

More questionable therapies include mesotherapy, a French technique where small amounts of various homeopathic solutions are injected beneath the surface of the skin to improve circulation and lymphatic and venous drainage. However, there are no scientific studies to date substantiating claims that mesotherapy eliminates cellulite or improves any other condition for which it is touted. Numerous herbal and dietary supplements claim to cure the internal causes of cellulite and speed up the metabolism. However, these nutraceutical supplements are not regulated by the FDA because they are not considered drugs, so industry claims do not have to be substantiated. The same goes for topical products that contain a variety of active ingredients including caffeine, green tea, DMAE, botanical extracts, retinol, and aminophylline (which is an asthma drug). Of these, retinoic acid can be used to strengthen the dermis, which represents your best bet for a topical formula. Many creams may improve the look of cellulite by hydrating and swelling the skin, but the effects are only temporary. Until reliable data is provided concerning any herbal or dietary remedy or topical therapy, as a physician, I cannot in good faith recommend these products to my patients.

Although there are some treatments that may provide temporary improvement in the appearance of cellulite, there is still no proven permanent cure for it. The lower body lift, however, can offer a definite improvement, although the surgery required is substantial. The lower body lift is a technique that requires an incision around the entire circumference of the abdominal area, so that excess skin is removed and the entire flank, thigh and buttocks areas can be lifted in one stage. The result of the procedure is tightening of the back, flank and abdominal tissues, and reduction in the appearance of cellulite in the lifted areas because the skin has been stretched. It is major surgery and definitely not for the weak of heart. It is rarely undertaken for the sole purpose of improving cellulite, but smoothed-out dimpling is an added benefit.

Breast Reshaping with Shorter Scars

Surgery on the breasts has been a primary focus of plastic surgeons since its advent. The number of articles published on breast surgery far exceeds all other areas of cosmetic and plastic surgery. Indeed, there are numerous techniques that have evolved

A vicious cycle is created: no exercise results in increasing weight gain, which results in increasing breast size.

since the late 1800s when breast reductions were initially performed. Plastic surgeons are always in pursuit of the perfect technique for reducing and lifting the breasts. However, the ultimate scarless technique has yet to be perfected.

Breast Reduction

Heavy, large, and pendulous breasts can cause substantial problems for women who are so endowed. Specifically, breast traction on the shoulders and spine can result in neck strain, headaches, back pain, poor posture, and skin inflammation underneath the breast mound. Numbness can be caused by the abnormal pressure of large breasts on the nerves that exit the arms. Women with large breasts are frequently overweight (in many cases to overcompensate for the abnormal proportions of their breasts). Many women, young and mature alike, curtail athletic activities to avoid the embarrassment and the additional strain and pain that large breasts cause during vigorous workouts. A vicious cycle is created: no exercise results in increasing weight gain, which results in increasing breast size. Breast reduction surgery can significantly improve the quality of life for many women with minimal emotional, physical, and financial costs. It is for this reason that breast reduction patients rank among the happiest in any plastic surgeon's office.

It is not surprising that many women seek relief from the symptoms related to their large breasts in hopes of attaining an aesthetically pleasant size, symmetry, and sensation. During the early- to mid-1900s, there were substantial improvements in the techniques used for breast lifts and reduction.

The most common methods for breast reduction involve a pedicle, or platform of tissue that is not excised so that nerve loss or areola necrosis is minimized. There are numerous variations of this technique that may be recommended, depending on the size of your breasts. Pedicle techniques are recommended for moderately large or heavy breasts. The surgeon removes excess breast tissue and skin while preserving a central breast mound. The nipple and areola are repositioned but remain attached to their blood and nerve supplies. The incisions are usually made under the crease of the breast, sometimes extending out to beneath the arm, around the nipple and areola, and vertically down from the nipple.

Women with large, pendulous breasts and thin, stretched skin may require a nipple graft technique. Because the nipple is so far from where the surgeon wants to place it, the nipple and areola are removed from the breast and grafted back onto the reduced breast. This procedure involves an anchor-shaped incision that circles the areola, extends downward, and follows the natural curve of the crease beneath the breast.

One of the most interesting breast reduction techniques to evolve is the use of liposuction alone to reduce breasts of moderate size. This can be done with a small puncture incision underneath the breast mound. It eliminates the need for the substantial scars that are typically required for larger breast reductions. This gives women who have been in the "gray zone" for breast reduction an opportunity to improve their breast shape and size with minimal scarring.

The recovery period for breast reduction surgery

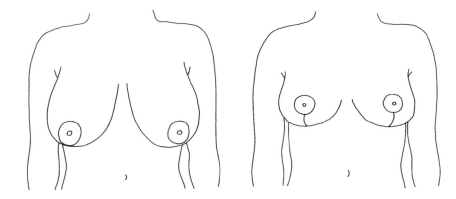

Breast Reduction

is surprisingly short. Most women will need to wear a bra for a minimum of one week after surgery to help diminish the risk of collection of blood or serum underneath the breasts by the compressive forces of the bra. Most patients are able to get back to vigorous activity within three weeks. It is common to lose substantial weight after surgery, as patients are frequently able to increase their athletic activity.

Most women are surprised to find how little pain they have after breast reduction surgery. It is not uncommon for patients to report that they used only one or two pain pills during their entire postoperative course. In fact, breast augmentation surgery is often substantially more painful than breast reduction due to manipulation of the underlying pectoralis major muscle. Breast reduction surgery is performed predominantly on the breast mound, which produces very little discomfort.

Another common misconception is that all breast lifts and reductions will result in loss of sensation in

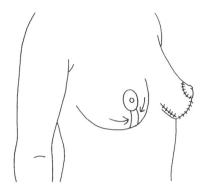

Classic Breast Lift Technique

the nipple and areolar area. While it is true that some women will lose sensation in the nipple, using some of the newer techniques of breast reduction, many women actually report improved sensation. The reason for this is that breast reduction diminishes traction on the sensory nerves to the nipple complex. Once the breast is made smaller, there is much less pull on the nerve that gives feeling to the nipple, and feeling improves in many patients.

Breast-feeding after breast reduction or lift surgery depends upon the technique used by the individual surgeon. Unless the breasts are extremely large requiring an extensive reduction, 50% of patients can go on to breast-feed. It is rare but possible that the nipple and areola may lose their blood supply and the tissue will suffer from necrosis and have to be treated while it heals.

Breast reduction scars can be extensive and permanent. They often remain lumpy and red for months, and then gradually fade to thin lines. Scars can often be placed inconspicuously so that patients can wear low-cut tops. For thickened or raised scars, I often recommend applying a silicone gel to speed healing. Another potential complication of large breast reductions that is more common with free nipple graft methods is the loss of pigment around the areola. This can be improved if necessary with micropigmentation or tattooing. The procedure can also leave slightly mismatched breasts or unevenly positioned nipples.

The goals of breast reduction surgery are to decrease the volume of the breasts while maintaining the sensitivity and blood supply to the nipple complex, and creating an esthetically pleasing breast contour with as minimal scarring as possible.

Breast Lifts

Over the years, gravity — along with pregnancy and nursing or substantial weight loss — can cause the breasts to sag. This is compounded by the loss in the skin of elastin and collagen, the chemical compounds that give all skin its elasticity.

A breast lift or mastopexy is a surgical procedure used to reshape sagging breasts. As with all areas of aesthetic surgery, the effects are not permanent, instead serving to turn back the clock rather than stopping it. Most women who seek a breast lift do so because pregnancy and nursing or weight fluctuations have left them with breasts that have been stretched due to increased breast volume and then reduced due to usual postpregnancy or weight loss changes. While breast tissue gets larger and smaller, the skin envelope which contains the breast tissue does not always bounce back after pregnancy or massive weight loss.

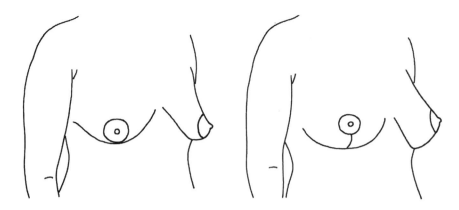

Vertical Breast Lift

Breast lifts are performed by creating an anchor-like incision on the breast. This leaves the patient with an incision around the areola, a vertical incision from the areola to the fold where the breast meets the chest, and an incision in the fold along the breast/chest margin. There are a variety of short-scar techniques that aim to eliminate the medial scar under the breast fold. In some cases, techniques can be used that eliminate the long vertical part of the scar. In most cases, the nipples remain attached to their blood vessels and nerves. Reduction of the breast with the vertical technique eliminates the inframammary scar. Although the ideal candidate for this technique has moderately large breasts and elastic skin, many surgeons apply modified scar techniques to all breast types.

Women over the age of 35 should have a baseline mammogram prior to any breast surgery. Most breast lifts and reductions are performed under general anesthesia, but this varies among

As with most scars, the final outcome cannot be seen for six months to one year after surgery.

surgeons. Surgery is performed as an outpatient procedure in either a hospital, an outpatient surgery center, or in an office-based accredited operating room facility.

After surgery, there is minimal pain and bruising. A surgical bra is worn around the clock after surgery for at least two to three weeks. Exercise can be started approximately one month after surgery. As with most scars, the final outcome cannot be seen for six months to one year after surgery. Massage will help scars to fade. Most women can usually wear the lowest-cut tops and bikinis, since the scars are placed in inconspicuous locations.

Possible complications associated with a breast lift include mild asymmetries, scars, and the potential for loss of sensation in the nipple areolar complex. If you are considering subsequent pregnancies, it is generally recommended that you postpone breast lift surgery until after your last pregnancy to minimize the affects of pregnancy on the final outcome.

In some cases, breast implants are needed to enhance the effects of the breast lift due to severe loss of breast volume. This can easily be done as a combined operation.

Breast Implants

On the surface, breast enlargement may seem like a straightforward concept. But it's not that simple. The truth is that breast augmentation requires great skill, precision, and experience for a successful outcome. Since I perform over 500 breast augmentations per year, our operating time is markedly reduced compared to the national average. This results in a very low incidence of complications and re-operations, and a faster recovery time for our patients.

Every woman considering breast implants is faced with several important decisions. No two breasts are exactly alike, and there are a variety of options to fit individual women's needs and anatomy. Making the right choices involves an extensive evaluation and honest discussion with a qualified plastic surgeon who can present all of your options. We believe strongly that the patient has to be involved in all stages of the process.

A breast augmentation procedure is usually performed in an outpatient surgical center under local anesthesia with intravenous sedation, or general anesthesia. General anesthesia may be chosen for women desiring implant placement below the muscle, since that procedure can be more uncomfortable. The surgery consists of making an incision, lifting the breast tissue, creating a pocket in the chest/breast area, and placing an envelope containing a soft implant material underneath. An incision may be made in any one of the following places: the crease below the breast, around the areola, under the armpit, through a concomitant tummy tuck incision, or through the navel, which is much less common. The implants can be placed either under the chest muscle or directly under the breasts. Placement considerations include the anatomy of your breasts, breast-feeding issues, your lifestyle, and personal preference. I strongly feel that most women should have implants placed under the muscle. This location yields better shape, better visualization of breast tissue on mammograms, less potential for hardening, and less rippling.

Incision
- Under the breast (inframammary)
- Around the nipple areola complex (periareolar)
- Under the armpit (transaxillary)
- Through the navel (transumbilical)
- Through a tummy tuck incision (transabdominoplasty)

Implant Texture
- Coated or textured
- Smooth

Implant Shape
- Round high profile; round low profile
- Teardrop

In the United States currently, only saline-filled implants are available for cosmetic use. However, based on the latest safety studies, silicone gel-filled implants will likely be available again soon.

Every woman should be considered on an individual basis. Skin quality and the amount of breast tissue factor into the decisions surrounding the best procedure for you. In my experience, most women are pleased with round implants, which are less expensive than teardrop-shaped implants. Teardrop implants are also more difficult to place and have a tendency to shift. My preference is for high-profile round implants; they have a lower rate of rippling and a natural look. Recent studies comparing mammograms of women with teardrop and round implants under the muscle indicate that in the body they are indistinguishable, due to the greater compression of the pectoral muscle at the top of the implant.

Textured implants have a thick coating which makes them feel harder for longer. The use of textured implants diminishes the risk of hardening of the breast, or capsular contracture. In our practice, the incidence of capsule formation is less then 1%. In the United States, there are four smooth implants used for every one textured. Smooth, round implants are the most forgiving and have a lower rate of complications.

Although it may seem that placing the breast implant scar under the armpit is more inconspicuous,

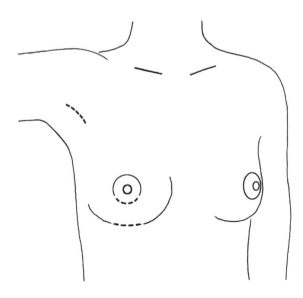

Breast Implant Incisions

you are more likely to go sleeveless than topless. An armpit incision can lead to unnecessary risks of the implant riding higher on the chest and potential re-operation. The most commonly used incision location for breast implants is under the breast, which is considered the gold standard because it is user friendly and predictable. Some women prefer to hide the incision around the nipple, which also heals nicely. It is also more common to place saline-filled implants underneath the chest muscle. The advantages of placing implants underneath the muscle include reduced chance of impaired mammography, a significantly lower risk of hardening of the tissue surrounding the implant, less rippling, and a more natural look and feel.

Breast implants are classified as a medical device, and all devices can fail over time. The average life expectancy of an implant is approximately 15 years, and the rate of deflation or rupture is only about 1% per year. Depending on the age at which you have your breasts enhanced, you can expect to have more than one pair of implants in your lifetime.

The Pros and Cons of Body Contouring

Liposuction is a versatile procedure for both women and men. With the face and chin area, including the neck and jowls, liposuction works well on younger people with resilient, elastic skin. It's a great way to forestall a face-lift; however, it doesn't always work as well after the mid-40s because skin shrinkage cannot be guaranteed.

Women with thicker skin and men in general have a better chance of skin contraction. Facial fat doesn't always need to be removed; it can be redistributed to fill in creases and hollows.

The upper extremities, including flabby upper arms and full forearms, can be trimmed down, along with the axillary folds, those flabby appendages that peek over your bra in the front and back. Even the fatty tissues of the breasts can be suctioned to reduce the size and heaviness of large breasts.

The upper and lower abdomen and waist are common key areas for liposuction. The upper back and back rolls that protrude around your bra straps and in bare dresses can be whittled down. The upper hips or flanks, often called "love handles" in men, also respond well to treatment. The banana rolls or flabby rolls under the buttocks can be slimmed. The outer or lateral thighs (also called the "saddle bags") and the inner thighs are perhaps the most popular and effective areas to treat. In heavy legs, the front and back of the thighs can also be suctioned to reduce the dimensions of the thighs. The inner knee can be made smaller, but this area is often a combination of cartilage, bone, and fat deposits so results may not be as dramatic. Even heavy calves and ankles can be recontoured with smaller instruments to produce a slimmer shape.

Liposuction

Suction-assisted lipectomy, also referred to as liposuction, is the most popular aesthetic surgery technique performed in the United States today. A common misconception about liposuction is that it is a quick-fix weight loss technique. In reality, this

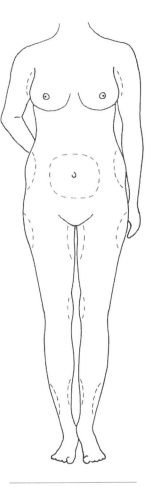

Liposuction is about shape, not weight. It is intended for people at or close to their ideal body weight with diet- or exercise-resistant fat deposits.

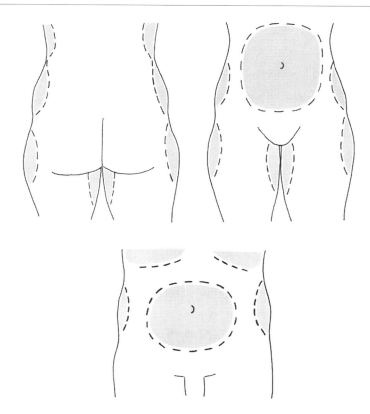

Typical Liposuction Areas for Women (top); Typical Male Areas (above).

is absolutely not the case. In our practice, approximately one-third of all people seeking liposuction are turned away as poor candidates for the procedure. Liposuction is a localized fat reduction technique for people with disproportionate areas of fat deposits. It is a wonderful method for removing fat that does not respond to honest attempts at diet and exercise, producing a more aesthetic, attractive contour. Most surgeons limit the amount of liposuction to five liters per session. This reduces the rate of risks and complications.

When cosmetic surgeons assess your body for liposuction, they focus on areas that are too full as well as areas that may be fat deficient. In order to achieve an ideal curve, we might need to transfer fat from one area and add it to a neighboring one in order to create an ideal silhouette, such as in the buttock region.

The best candidates for liposuction are of relatively normal weight and have firm skin with good elastic rebound. The more elastic the skin, the better liposuction works. If you have flabby skin due to pregnancies, aging, or weight fluctuations, liposuction can potentially make it look worse.

Unfortunately, anyone with a significant amount of stretch marks or loose skin will require additional surgical procedures to remove excess skin which will leave visible scars. Patients who have significant underlying medical problems such as diabetes or poor blood supply to the extremities are not good candidates for this procedure. Cellulite also does not respond to liposuction, even though liposuction will make you look slimmer.

There are some possible risks and complications associated with liposuction. Major risks include infection, hemorrhage or bleeding, post-operative asymmetries, which could require subsequent touch-ups, dimpling of the skin, and fat or blood clots which could travel to the lungs, causing respiratory or breathing problems. The scars from liposuction are usually small, about one-quarter inch, and are placed strategically to minimize their appearance. They are usually placed in the bikini line or belly button or other inconspicuous areas.

Tumescent liposuction. The new technique associated with liposuction is referred to as tumescent liposuction ("tumescent" means distention). By injecting large amounts of saline solution mixed with a blood vessel constricting agent known as adrenaline, blood loss and postoperative bruising are dramatically lowered. The added benefit of tumescent liposuction is that by adding a Lidocaine or Novocaine solution to the mix, the procedure can be done relatively comfortably while the patient is under only mild sedation.

Ultrasound-assisted lipoplasty. Ultrasonic sound waves, like shock waves, are transmitted into the fatty tissues from the tip of the cannula probe. The fat cells are melted or liquefied and then removed by low-pressure vacuum through a suction tube. Ultrasonic liposuction is often reserved for large volumes and multiple areas, as well as more difficult areas to contour where the deep fat is thicker, more fibrous and harder to extract (ie, back rolls, upper abdomen, and flanks). It is usually combined with traditional liposuction when both the deeper fat and more superficial fat are being removed. When previous liposuction has been done, it may be useful to soften the scar tissue that develops to make it easier for the surgeon to extract the fat. External ultrasound waves in lower frequencies can also be used with liposuction to soften fat deposits from the skin's surface, although this practice is controversial.

Power-assisted lipoplasty. One of the latest advances in liposuction technology is the addition of power. The cannulas (tubular instruments used in liposuction to remove fat) are motor-driven so they vibrate, which makes removing fat easier and faster for the surgeon. The primary advantage is that there is less physical exertion required for the surgeon to remove the fat with this method.

Vaser®-assisted lipoplasty. The Vaser system utilizes probes with a grooved design and continuous bursts of ultrasonic vibrational energy to selectively target larger fat cells which are then removed by suction.

The postoperative period after liposuction has a modest amount of pain associated with it. You will be instructed to wear a girdle or compression garment for a minimum of three to six weeks after the operation. This enhances the outcome of surgery by compressing the tunnels that were created during the operation. Most liposuction is now done successfully on an outpatient basis. The immediate postoperative period is associated with some bruising. All patients who undergo liposuction will be firm and lumpy for several weeks after surgery and it takes approximately three to six months to see the final outcome.

The rippling we used to see with liposuction several years ago has been substantially reduced by using smaller diameter cannulas. The reduced-diameter cannulas associated with tumescent liposuction have also dramatically improved the safety and quality of this procedure.

Patient satisfaction from properly performed lipo-suction is overwhelmingly positive. In my experience, it is rare to find a patient who isn't thrilled with the results when the procedure is performed properly.

Tummy Tucks

Abdominoplasty, also known as "tummy tuck," is a cosmetic operation done to remove excess skin and fat from the abdomen and flank area. The procedure is useful for men or women who are bothered by large fat deposits or loose skin that does not respond to diet or exercise. It is very helpful for women who have had one or more children and who have lax lower abdominal musculature. Additionally, in those patients who have sustained massive weight loss, loose, hanging skin can be a problem that can be treated in no other fashion.

Tummy tuck or abdominoplasty surgery should be undertaken in those patients who are near their

---

Three Approaches to Abdomen Contouring

- For some patients, liposuction of the abdomen alone will produce a thin abdominal wall and flank region.
- For those patients who have laxity and excess skin below their belly button, a mini tummy tuck is all that is necessary.
- For those patients who have significant laxity of their abdominal musculature or who have excess skin, a formal tummy tuck is the only way to achieve improvement.

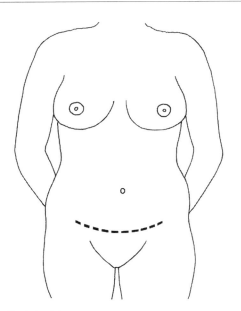

Mini Tuck Incision

ideal weight through diet or exercise. It can be safely combined with many other operations, including breast reduction, augmentation, or liposuction of other areas in the body.

There are three different approaches to contouring your abdomen. The approach chosen by your surgeon will depend on your goals and your specific anatomic problems.

A mini tummy tuck involves a smaller incision in the bikini area and no incision around the belly button. Through this incision, excess skin and fat are removed, usually in association with liposuction of the upper abdominal wall and flank region. Permanent sutures are then placed into the abdominal musculature to tighten the abdominal wall. Excess skin and fat are resected and the wound is closed.

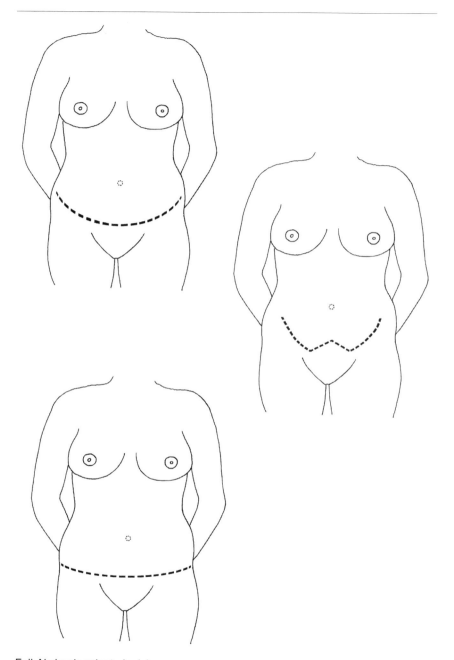

Full Abdominoplasty Incisions

In those patients who have significant excess skin throughout their abdominal wall or laxity of the entire abdominal musculature, a full tummy tuck is done. This involves an incision around the belly button, as well as a somewhat longer hip-to-hip scar. Through this incision, the entire abdominal wall is surgically tightened with permanent sutures. Excess skin and fat are removed and the belly button is brought out through a separate incision in the abdominal wall. The surgical site also involves the placement of plastic drain tubes. These remain in place for five to seven days after surgery and are relatively painless to remove. Patients are required to wear some form of girdle or abdominal binder after surgery for three to four weeks to achieve maximum benefit. Exercise should be delayed for four to six weeks after surgery. Most patients are back to work in seven to 14 days after the operation.

As with all operations, tummy tuck surgery has some risks. The major risks are infection and scars around the belly button and in the lower bikini region. Indeed, the scars can be quite conspicuous, but the trade-off is a better contoured, flatter abdomen. It will take nine months to a year before those scars flatten, soften, and fade. Additionally, tummy tuck surgery has been associated with blood clots in the legs, which can cause lung problems. Collection of fluid underneath the surgery site is common after tummy tuck surgery and will frequently require several episodes of drainage. Fortunately, this is not a difficult problem to contend with and is not painful for the patient.

Most patients will have numbness around the abdomen, which can last up to one year. Some

The next step up from tummy tucks is a body lift. A body lift is ideal for patients who have had significant weight loss and have been left with unsightly loose pouches of excess skin.

patients never regain full sensation in the area of the surgery. Alterations are often seen in the appearance of the patient's belly button after tummy tuck surgery and this is typically permanent. The risks of wound problems are always present with tummy tuck surgery and the problems with wound healing increase in those patients who smoke and in those patients who have had incisions in their abdomen from other operations. This is particularly true for patients who have had upper abdominal incisions, which are placed in the horizontal direction, such as a prior gallbladder surgical incision.

The next step up from tummy tucks is a body lift. A body lift is ideal for patients who have had significant weight loss and have been left with unsightly loose pouches of excess skin. It is the most effective technique to restore firm, youthful contours to the body. Lower body lifts can address the thighs, buttocks, abdomen, waist, and hips all in one stage. The added benefits are an overall improvement in dimpling and cellulite. The trade-off is that the recovery period is longer than those of other cosmetic surgical procedures, and the length of the scarring is significant.

Abdominoplasty surgery can be performed as an in- or outpatient procedure, and can be done under general or spinal anesthesia. Results can be dramatic, creating a narrower waist and a long-lasting, trim figure.

In a brachioplasty, or arm lift, the scars are placed from elbow to armpit and can be rather conspicuous. In my practice, this surgery is reserved for the most severe cases of hanging arm skin, due to the unsightly nature of the ensuing scars.

Glossary

A

abdominoplasty — Plastic surgery of the abdomen in which excess fatty tissue and skin are removed.

ablation — Vaporization of the most superficial layers of skin.

acne — A chronic skin condition characterized by an inflammatory eruption of the skin that occurs when a hair follicle gets plugged with sebum and dead cells. Rising hormone levels stimulate oil glands, which cause clogged pores and inflammation.

actinic keratosis — (Solar keratosis) a lesion that is dry, scaly, rough, and tan or pink caused by sun exposure, considered precancerous.

alar base — The wing-like structures at the base of the nose.

alkaline — A nonacid substance with a pH greater than seven.

allantoin — A botanical extract said to heal and soothe. Used in creams and topical preparations for the skin.

allergen — A substance that can cause allergic reaction.

allograft — A graft from the same species as the recipient, as in human skin.

alopecia — A condition of hair loss.

alpha hydroxy acid — (AHA) A group of acids derived from foods such as fruit and milk, which can improve the texture of the skin by removing layers of dead cells and encouraging cell regeneration. There are many AHAs but the most common forms are lactic acid, glycolic acid, pyruvic acid, tartaric acid and maleic acid.

anatomic breast implant — Teardrop-shaped implant as opposed to the round style, designed to look more like a natural breast.

anemia — A pathological deficiency in the oxygen-carrying component of the blood, measured in unit volume concentrations of hemoglobin, red blood cell volume, or red blood cell number.

antioxidant — A substance designed to prevent a chemical reaction with oxygen, eg, vitamins C, E, A, grape seed, green tea.

areola — The pigmented skin around the nipple.

arnica — A botanical derived from a mountain plant with antiseptic, astringent, antimicrobial, and anti-inflammatory properties.

autologous — Occurring naturally in a certain type of tissue of the body.

B

banana roll — The "roll" of fat directly situated beneath the buttock crease.

benzoyl peroxide — An antibacterial ingredient commonly used to treat acne.

beta HCG — human chorionic gonadotropin. The "pregnancy hormone" is produced by the placenta.

beta hydroxy acid (salicylic acid) — A family of acids that enhance cell renewal, found naturally in willow bark.

bioactive — Substances that achieve cosmetic results by some degree of physiological action, eg, fruit acids.

bleaching agents — Substances which slow down or block the production of melanin to lighten age spots and fade areas of hyperpigmentation; ie, hydroquinone, kojic acid, azelaic acid.

blepharitis — Inflammation of the eyelids, characterized by redness and swelling and dried crusts.

blepharoplasty (eyelid plasty) — Surgery to remove excess fat, muscle, and/or skin around the eyes. Incisions follow the natural contour lines of the upper and lower lids, or can be done through the lining of the lower eyelid, providing access to skin and fatty issue.

body lift — The procedure involves liposuction of any excess fat in the thighs and legs, then removing excess skin high up on the outer thighs and above the buttocks, loosening the tissues below this and pulling them up and suturing them together. Deep stitches are secured to the ligaments and bone and the length of the incision is determined by the amount of excess skin to be removed.

botanical — Refers to products derived from plants.

Botulinium toxin — A naturally occurring toxin that is injected into facial muscles to temporarily paralyze them and eliminate expression lines of the face, around the eyes, and the neck.

brachioplasty — An arm lift involving placing an incision in the armpit and continuing towards the inside of the elbow to remove primarily excess skin and fat from the upper arm and recontour the arms.

buffer — An additive that adjusts the pH balance of a skin preparation.

buccal fat pads — Fat pads located in the cheek, also known as the fat pad of Bichet.

C

cannulas — Long, thin hollow tubular instrument used to extract fat during liposuction.

capillary — The smallest type of blood vessel in the body. Spider veins, for instance, are actually small capillaries commonly found on the face or legs.

capsular contracture — Scar tissue that forms in the pocket surrounding a breast implant and becomes hardened and distorted.

carbon dioxide — Laser technology that can be used to resurface moderate to deep facial wrinkles, scars, and can also be used as a cutting tool.

cauterize — To burn or sear abnormal tissue with a cautery or caustic instrument, such as a laser.

cellulite — Deposits of fat, toxins and fluids trapped in pockets beneath the skin, more common in women.

cheek-lift — See midface-lift.

chemical peel — A procedure in which a solution of varying strengths is applied to the entire face or to specific areas, such as around the mouth, to peel away the skin's top layers. Common peeling agents are alpha hydroxy acid, beta hydroxy acid, trichloracetic acid (TCA), Jessner's solution, and phenol.

coenzyme Q10 — A renewal agent that stimulates natural cell energy production and regenerates vitamin E.

collagen — A primary component of human skin that gives it resiliency, suppleness and tone, and breaks down with age due to muscle movement and environmental damage.

collagenase — Enzyme that breaks down collagen.

columella — The strip of skin dividing the nostrils at the base of the nose.

comedones — Open (blackheads) and closed (whiteheads) formed when pores become clogged with natural oils and impurities.

commissure — The area where two anatomic parts meet, as in the corner of the eye or the lips, typically referring to a fold or crease.

computer imaging — The use of a computer enhanced image to allow a doctor or dentist to illustrate how you may look after treatment, used as a patient education tool.

congenital defect — Abnormality formed at birth.

coronal — Of or pertaining to the top of the head or skull.

corrugator — Muscle that is responsible for causing the glabellar or vertical lines that form between the eyebrows.

cosmeceutical — A substance that falls between the classification of a drug and a cosmetic, ie, nonprescription over-the-counter formulations that provide pharmaceutical benefits.

craniofacial surgery — Surgery of the face and head.

crust — Surface layer formed by the drying of a bodily secretion.

D

deflation — A rupture or tear in the shell of a breast implant that causes the filler (saline, silicone gel, or other) to leak out and the implant to flatten.

dehiscence — A rupture or splitting open, as of a surgical wound, or of an organ or structure to discharge its contents.

dermabrasion — Nonsurgical resurfacing procedure in which a hand-held rotary wheel is used to remove the top layer of skin.

dermal fillers — A category of substances that are either injected or implanted to shape and form overlying tissue.

dermatitis — An inflammatory condition of the skin that is characterized by itching and redness. Three categories of dermatitis are atopic, contact and seborrheic.

dermis — The layer of skin composed of collagen and elastin, lying beneath the epidermis (outer layer) and above the subcutaneous layers.

diode — Contact laser technology that cuts and coagulates tissue.

dorsum — The upper, outer surface of an organ, as in the nose.

dry eye — A condition of the eyelids which causes dryness, blurred vision and the eyes to feel gritty.

E

ecchymosis — The passage of blood from ruptured blood vessels into subcutaneous tissue, marked by a purple discoloration of the skin.

echinacea — A natural substance thought to boost the immune system, and have antiitching and soothing properties.

ectropion — A condition of the lower eyelid in which the lid is pulled downward from loose eyelid skin, muscles or too much skin having been removed, also called "lid retraction".

eczema — A chronic skin condition that superficial inflation in areas of the skin and scalp.

elastin — A protein that is similar to collagen and the chief constituent of elastic fibers, also used as a surface protective agent in cosmetics to alleviate dry skin.

electrolysis — Use of electric current to permanently destroy the hair's root bulb.

endoscopic surgery — An endoscope is a small rigid tube-like instrument equipped with fiberoptic lighting, which can be introduced into the body through a tiny incision so that it lights up the surgical area. The surgeon can see the area on a video monitor while performing an operation, as in endoscopic brow lifting, breast augmentation, face-lifting and tummy tucks.

electrocautery — To burn tissue with an electric current by use of a specially designed apparatus.

electromyograph — An instrument used in the diagnosis of neuromuscular disorders that produces an audio or visual record of the electrical activity of a skeletal muscle by means of an electrode inserted into the muscle or placed on the skin.

electromyography — The diagnosis of neuromuscular disorders with the use of an electromyograph.

encapsulation — The act of inclosing in a capsule; the growth of a membrane around (any part) so as to enclose it in a capsule.

endoscopic — Pertaining to an endoscope, an instrument for visualizing the interior of a hollow organ.

epidermis — The outermost layer of the skin.

epidural blocks — Regional anesthesia resulting from injection of an anesthetic into the epidural space of the spinal cord; sensation is lost in the abdominal and genital and pelvic areas; used in childbirth and gynecological surgery.

epinephrine — A white to brownish crystalline compound isolated from the adrenal glands of certain mammals or synthesized and used in medicine as a heart stimulant, vasoconstrictor, and bronchial relaxant.

epithelialization— Regeneration of the epithelium or superficial layer of the skin, as occurs after laser resurfacing.

erbium:YAG — A type of ablative laser that produces energy in a wavelength that penetrates the skin, is readily absorbed by water (a major component of tissue cells), and scatters the heat effects of the laser light.

erythema — Redness of the skin, as in post laser or other resurfacing, etc.

exfoliate — A material that removes dead surface skin cells.

exfoliation — To remove a layer of skin in flakes; peel.

external ultrasound —Utilizing ultrasonic energy applied externally to the skin to dissolve or liquefy fat deposits prior to liposuction.

extrusion — The erosion of skin that causes an implant (chin, lip, breast, etc.) to become partially exposed.

F

face-lift: See **rhytidectomy**

fascia — The sheet of connective tissue that covers the muscles, sometimes used as a graft material.

fat embolus — Globules of fat that can infiltrate the bloodstream during surgery causing a mass that can result in serious complication and death.

fibrin sealant — A natural agent for the achievement of rapid hemostasis and tissue sealing in a variety of surgical applications, also referred to as tissue glue.

fibroblast — A cell from which connective tissue develops.

filler — A category of substances that are either injected or implanted to shape and form overlying tissue. Common fillers are bovine collagen, the patient's own fat or collagen from skin, human donor collagen.

follicle — A sheath that surrounds the root of the hair.

forehead lift — Also called a brow-lift, pulls up droopy brows and upper lids, and improves wrinkling and vertical and horizontal frown lines. The open forehead lift is more invasive than the endoscopic brow-lift. An "open" means that you will have an incision placed at or behind the ear through which excess skin is removed and muscles are tightened. An "endoscopic" lift employs three to five tiny incisions (one-half inch to one inch) placed behind the hairline to remove muscles that cause frowning and wrinkles and/or elevate your brows.

free radicals — A destructive form of oxygen generated by each cell in the body that destroys cellular membranes.

frontalis — The muscle that enables the brows to move up and down, and contributes to the formation of horizontal wrinkles of the forehead.

G

general anesthesia — Commonly referred to as "being asleep," a total loss of consciousness is induced by an anesthetist or anesthesiologist. The patient doesn't feel anything, and a breathing tube is placed in the airway.

genioplasty — To add projection to the chin, the bones are broken so that the chin area can be moved forward and secured in place.

glabella — The area between the eyebrows in the center of the forehead where deep vertical lines and creases often develop.

graft — A piece of tissue that is totally removed from one part of the body and transferred to another area of the body, as in fat, cartilage, bone, skin, etc.

glaucoma — Any of a group of eye diseases characterized by abnormally high intraocular fluid pressure, damaged optic disk, hardening of the eyeball, and partial to complete loss of vision.

glycerin — Used in moisturizers due to its water binding capabilities.

glycolic acid — an organic substance, found naturally in unripe grapes and in the leaves of the wild grape, and produced artificially in many ways, as by the oxidation of glycol.

gynecomastia — Male breast reduction procedure, usually accomplished via liposuction through small incisions in the areola and/or chest wall.

H

hematoma — A localized accumulation of blood in the skin caused by a blood vessel wall rupture, possible complication of surgery that may have to be drained.

hyaluronic acid — An acid found naturally in the body and helps retain the skin's natural moisture.

hydroquinone — A bleaching agent that slows down or blocks the production of melanin to lighten age spots and to fade darkness and blotchiness.

hyperpigmentation — Darkening of certain skin areas through overproduction of melanin.

hypertrophic scar — Thickened, raised, or red scar tissue.

hypertrophy — Enlarged or thickened area

hypoallergenic — A substance with a low chance of causing allergy or skin irritation.

hypopigmentation — Reduction in the pigment cells in the skin resulting in skin lightening.

hypoplasia — Incomplete or arrested development of an organ or a part.

I

inframammary crease — The skin crease or fold that lies beneath the breast.

inframammary — Below the mammary gland.

intense pulsed light therapy — A broad spectrum of light that produces results on age spots and broken capillaries and is used to treat full face, neck, chest or hands.

isolagen — Autologous filler fashioned from collagen from your own skin that is grown in a laboratory; processed and liquefied for later injection into wrinkles and folds.

J

jaw — Used to describe the maxillae and mandible and soft tissue surrounding the bony structure.

Jessner's solution — Pronounced "yes-nerz," a pre-measured solution formulated with resorcinol, salicylic acid, lactic acid with ethanol originally developed by Dr. Max Jessner at New York University Hospital for the treatment of acne.

K

keloid — Enlarged, permanent and thickened scar formations that are more common in darker skin types, and often run in families.

keratin — A surface protective agent with film-forming and moisturizing action.

kinetin — Compound of N-6-furfuryladenine, a synthetic plant growth factor.

kojic acid — Natural skin-lightening agent derived from a Japanese mushroom.

L

lactic acid — A component of the skin's natural moisturizing factor.

lagopthalmus — Upper eyelid retraction that results in difficulty closing the upper eyelids.

L-ascorbic acid — The purest form of vitamin C, which when applied topically is an antioxidant, antiirritant, antiinflammatory.

laser — A device that amplifies light frequency radiation within or near the range of visible light. Name derived from acronym l(ight) a(mplification by) s(timulated) e(mission of) r(adiation).

lateral hooding — Excess fold of skin between the eyebrow and the outer portion of the upper eyelid.

lentigo — Benign tan or brown colored lesion on the skin from sun exposure.

lidocaine — A local anesthetic (trade name Xylocaine) used topically on the skin and mucous membranes.

local anesthesia — Medications (usually in the "caine" family) that are injected into a surgical or treatment site to cause temporary localized numbness.

lymphatic system — A network of structures, including ducts and nodes, that carry lymph fluid from tissues to the bloodstream.

M

malar bags — The pouch of loose skin and fluid that sometimes occurs with age below the lower eyelid area.

malar fat pad — A structure that sits in the second layer of the face below the cheekbone that is frequently positioned during facial rejuvenation procedures.

malarplasty — Cheekbone reduction or augmentation.

malic acid — A glycolic acid derived from apples.

mammogram — An x-ray image of the breast produced by mammography.

mandible — Jaw bone.

marionette lines — The vertical creases that form in the corners of the mouth towards the jowls.

mastopexy — Breast lift procedure performed to reshape the breast with or without nipple repositioning.

melanin — The pigment that gives skin its color.

melanoma — The deadliest form of skin cancer, characterized by a black or dark brown pigmented tumor.

mentoplasty — Plastic surgery of the chin whereby its shape or size is altered.

microdermabrasion — Also referred to as "derma-peeling" or "microabrasion" is a mechanical blasting of the face with sterile microparticles that abrade or rub off the very top skin layer, then vacuuming out the particles and the dead skin.

microabrasion — A tooth-whitening procedure using an abrasive combined with a hydrochloric acid.

midface-lift — Also referred to as a "cheek lift," a surgical procedure designed to lift sagging areas in the mid-face, including around the cheekbone areas below the eyes.

midline — An imaginary vertical line that divides the face or body into two equal areas.

milia — Tiny skin cysts that resemble whiteheads.

mitral valve prolapse — Cardiopathy resulting from the mitral valve not regulating the flow of blood between the left atrium and left ventricle of the heart.

Moh's surgery — Moh's surgery is typically used in skin cancer treatment. It results in a significantly smaller surgical defect and less-noticeable scarring as compared to other methods. The Moh's procedure is recommended for anatomic areas where maximum preservation of healthy tissue is desireable for cosmetic purposes, such as the face. It may also be indicated for lesions that have the greatest propensity for recurrence.

monitored anesthesia care — Also called "local with intravenous sedation" and "twilight," where medications are given intravenously to induce a state of sleepiness and relieve pain, supplemented with local anesthetic injections.

musculature — The system or arrangement of muscles in a body or a body part.

N

nasal labial folds — The region of the face between the nose and the corners of the lip, commonly referred to as "smile lines."

nasion — The depression at the root of the nose that indicates the junction where the forehead ends and the bridge of the nose begins.

necrosis — Dead skin cells.

nonablative laser resurfacing — A new class of lasers that does not produce a deep burn and provides a much less invasive treatment.

noncomedogenic — Products that are formulated not to clog the pores and cause pimples.

O

orbicularis oculi — The muscular body of the eyelid encircling the eye and comprising the palpebral, orbital, and lacrimal muscles. The palpebral muscle functions to close the eyelid gently; the orbital muscle functions to close it more energetically, such as in winking.

orbit — The cavity in the skull where the eyeballs, eye muscles, nerves and blood vessels rest.

osteotomy — The operation of dividing a bone or of cutting a piece out of it.

otoplasty — Reparative or plastic surgery of the auricle of the ear.

outpatient surgery — Ambulatory surgery in which you are discharged later the same day from the recovery room in a hospital, office surgical suite, or clinic.

P

PABA — Para aminobenzoic acid. Found in the vitamin B complex, used as an ingredient in some sunscreen products.

pectoralis — The muscle that is located between the rib cage and the chest tissue.

pectus excavatum — A congenital deformity of the pectus or chest, more popularly known as "funnel chest" or "sunken chest."

petrolatum — Used in creams, it softens and soothes skin. Forms a film to prevent moisture loss.

pH — The degree of acidity or alkalinity in the solution of products.

periareolar — The area around the areola.

periodontal disease — A disease that attacks the gum and bone and around the teeth.

phenol — Peeling formula applied to the skin to lighten pigment, soften wrinkles, and improve scars, considered to be a deep and more invasive peel.

phlebitis — Inflammation of a vein.

photoaging — Damage to the skin due to cumulative exposure to the sun; ie wrinkles, age spots, fine lines.

photosensitivity — Chemicals or topical ingredients that cause the skin to be reactive when exposed to sunlight such as inflammation, hyper-pigmentation and swelling.

platysma — A thin sheet of muscle located just beneath the skin of the chin and neck.

platysmal bands — Vertical strands of the muscle of the neck that can become more prominent with age and are often sutured or tightened during a face or neck lift.

polysaccharide — Any of a class of carbohydrates, such as starch and cellulose, consisting of a number of monosaccharides joined by glycosidic bonds.

pore — Small opening of the sweat glands of the skin.

procerus — Muscle that works with the corrugator muscles and contributes to the vertical frown lines between the eyebrows.

psoriasis — A noncontagious inflammatory skin disease characterized by recurring reddish patches covered with silvery scales.

ptosis — Pronounced "toe-sis," a term for drooping as in eyelids, breasts and brows.

pulmonary embolus — A blockage of an artery in the lungs by fat, air, tumor tissue, or blood clot.

R

rectus — Any of various straight muscles, such as, the abdomen, eye, neck, and thigh.

resorcinol — In mild solutions, used as an antiseptic and as a soothing preparation for itchy skin.

Retin-A® (tretinoin) — A topical medication derived from vitamin A that is used to treat photoaging and acne.

retinol — A gentler nonprescription strength alternative to retinoic acid. Retinol is an active form of vitamin A that works deep under the surface of the skin to visibly reduce lines and wrinkles.

rhytidectomy (face-lift) — Surgical procedure which rejuvenates the face by tightening the underlying musculature, removing excess fat deposits, and redraping sagging skin of the lower face and neck. Incisions are placed in the hairline and around the ears and/or under the chin.

rosacea — A common skin condition of the face, nose, cheeks, forehead that results in redness, pimples, dilated blood vessels, and occasional pustules.

S

saline — Salt water commonly used as a filler for breast implants and in the course of administering intravenous fluids.

Schirmer's test — A test that assesses tear production in the eyes and is helpful in treating dry eye syndrome.

scleral show — Lower eyelid retraction, which exposes the sclera (white part of the eyeball), below the pupil.

sclerotherapy — The injection of one of several solutions through a small needle directly into a vein to cause it to collapse.

sepsis — A reaction of the body to bacteria that circulate in the blood, characterized by chills and fever.

septoplasty — An operation to straighten the midline cartilage structure of the nose in order to improve breathing.

septum — The separating wall in the nose between the left and right nasal passages.

seroma — A collection of clear fluid that may occur under the skin following surgery.

silastic sheeting — Patches or strips of silicone that may be applied to the skin for extended time periods to soften and reduce scarring.

silastic — A sac made of rubber and silicone, often filled with silicone or salt solution.

silicone — A synthetic substance used in a gel-like form in silicone breast implants, in a liquid injectable form for facial areas, and in other medical devices.

SMAS — The superficial musculoaponeurotic system (SMAS), is a layer of tissue that covers the deeper structures in the cheek area and touches the superficial muscle covering the lower face and neck called the platysma. The SMAS is often lifted and repositioned during the face-lift procedure.

SPF (Sun Protection Factor) — A scale used to rate the level of protection sunscreens provide from UVB rays of the sun.

spider veins (telangiectasias) — Dilated or broken blood vessels near the surface of the skin.

spinal blocks — A form of anesthesia that numbs the lower two-thirds of the body.

steroids — Any of a large number of hormonal substances with similar basic chemical structure, produced mainly in the adrenal cortex and gonads.

stratum corneum — Surface layer of epidermis.

striae — Commonly known as stretch marks, caused by thinning of the underlying skin layer (dermis) that appear first as red, raised lines, then darken and flatten gradually to form shiny whitened streaks.

subglandular — Under the gland, typically of the breast.

submental — Referring to the area below the chin.

subpectoral — Also called submuscular, referring to the area below the pectoralis muscle where a breast implant may be placed.

subperiosteal — A term for a procedure that goes deep into multiple layers; a lift in which all tissues are separated from the underlying bone structure, thereby considered more invasive, as in brow, face, etc.

suction assisted lipectomy (liposuction) — A procedure in which localized collections of fat are removed from the face and/or body by using a high vacuum device through small incisions.

sunblock — A physical sunscreen or a barrier against the sun's ultraviolet rays. Available in creams or ointments.

suture — The fine thread or other material used surgically to close a wound or join tissues.

T

tartaric acid — A type of glycolic acid derived from apples.

tazarotene — A prescription topical retinoid (vitamin A derivative) approved for treating mild to moderate plaque psoriasis and photoaging.

tiplasty — A nose augmentation or reduction procedure concerning primarily the nasal tip.

tissue engineering — The science of production of human tissue *ex vivo* (outside of the human body), as in growing cartilage in tissue culture.

tissue glue — A compound used instead of stitches or staples in surgery.

titanium dioxide — A nonchemical, common agent used in sunscreen products that works by physically blocking the sun. It may be used alone or in combination with other agents.

tocopherol — Chemical name for vitamin E, an antioxidant.

tram flap — Acronym for "transverse rectus abdominis myocutaneous," a breast reconstruction method whereby a flap of abdominal fat and skin is moved to the chest wall to form a newly reconstructed breast.

tragus — A small extension of the auricular cartilage of the ear, anterior to the external meatus.

transaxillary — An incision placed under the arm for access during surgery, as in breast augmentation.

transumbilical — An approach whereby the incision is placed in the umbilicus (belly button) through which breast implants may be moved into position.

tretinoin — A derivative of vitamin A.

trichloroacetic acid — A colorless, deliquescent,

corrosive, crystalline compound, used topically as an astringent and antiseptic.

tumescent — A method of anesthesia where large volumes of local anesthetic and saline solution are injected to swell the area to be operated on, commonly used in liposuction and body contouring procedures.

twilight anesthesia — See monitored anesthesia care.

t-zone — The area of the face that consists of the forehead, nose, and the area around the mouth, including the chin.

U

ultrasound — Application of a sound wave, a mechanical vibration of more than 16,000 cycles per second.

umbilicus — Belly button or navel.

undermining — Surgical separation of tissues from their underlying structures.

UVA — Long wavelengths emitted by the sun which take longer to produce a burn than UVB but penetrate deeper into the skin to cause sun damage.

UVB — Short wavelengths emitted by the sun, which are known to cause premature aging and skin cancer.

V

varicose veins — Enlarged, dilated veins just below the surface of the skin, commonly found in the legs, caused by the valves becoming filled with blood.

vector — The direction of pull, as in face-lifting, etc.

vermillion border — The external pinkish-to-red area of the upper and lower lips. It extends from the junction of the lips with surrounding facial skin on the exterior to the labial mucosa within the mouth.

W

wavelength — The distance between a given point on one wave cycle and the corresponding point on the next successive wave cycle, the light of the wavelength produces a pure color.

witch's chin — Pointy or droopy chin syndrome.

X

xanthoma — A fatty deposit in the skin that may appear on the lower eyelids or elsewhere.

Y

YAG — Abbreviation for yttrium aluminate garnet, a crystal used in some types of lasers.

Z

zinc oxide — Chemical ingredient that has soothing and astringent qualities that can block ultraviolet rays of the sun.

Z-plasty — A z-shaped incisional technique used to conceal a scar in the natural skin creases.

zygomatic arch — An arch formed by the temporal process of the zygomatic bone with the zygomatic process of the temporal bone. The tendon of the temporal muscle passes beneath it.

Index

Garlic, 4, 127
GHK, 26
Gingko biloba, 127
Ginseng, 127
Glabellar creases, 75
Glutiathione peroxidase, 4
Glycerin, 38, 83
Glycoaminoglycosans, 13
Glycolic acid, 22, 28, 59, 60, 91, 95
    delivery to skin, 23
    formulation concentrations, 23
    mechanism of, 22
Glycolic peel, 130
Glycyl-L-histidyl-L-lysine (see GHK)
Glyquin, 59, 60
Glyquin XM Cream, 59
Gore-Tex, 89, 119
Granulomas, 84
Grapeseed extract, 32
Grapeseed oil, 38
Green tea, 32
Growth factors, 21, 29
    sources of, 29

Hair follicles, 47
Hair removal, 95
Hairline, 109
Hawthorn, 32
Headaches, 125
Heart murmur, 127
Hemangiomas, 95
Hematoma, 114
Hepatitis B core
    antibody (HBcAB), 80
Hepatitis B surface
    antigen (HBsAG), 80
Hepatitis C antibody (AntiHCV), 80
Herbal supplements, 127
High blood pressure, 125
High-intensity light technology, 96
Hip replacement, 127
Home peels, 94
    for oily skin, 94
Homeopathic solutions, 138
Hormones, 125
Human immunodeficiency
    virus antibody (antiHIV 1-2), 80
Human T-lymphotropic virus
    type I antibody (antiHTLV-1), 80
Humectants, 38
Hyaluronic acid, 38, 76, 77
Hyaluronic acid gels, 81
    injection of, 81
Hyaluronidase, 32
Hydration, 15
Hydroquinone, 28, 58, 59, 130
Hydroxy acid, 18
Hylaform, 82

Hyperpigmentation, 14, 46, 55, 56, 58, 62, 73, 92, 94, 95
    in pregnancy, 57
Hyperthyroidism, 109
Hypertrophic scars, 63
Hypopigmentation, 92, 100

Ibuprofen, 126
Immune system, 4
Intense pulsed light, 54, 61, 96, 98, 99, 135, 137
Intravenous sedation, 92
IPL (see intense pulsed light)
Irritability, 125
Isotretinoin, 52

Jessner's solution, 91
Joint replacement, 127
Jojoba oil, 38
Jowling, 114
Jowls, 104

Keloids, 63, 127
Keratin, 9
Keratinocyte growth factor, 29
Keratinocytes, 57
KGF (see keratinocyte growth factor)
Kinerase, 25
Kinetin, 25
    antioxidant properties of, 25
Kligman's formula, 130
Kojic acid, 28, 59, 61

Lactic acid, 24, 38, 59, 60, 91
    as exfoliant, 24
Lanolin, 38
Laparoscopy, 110
L-ascorbic acid, 26
Lasers, 44, 95
    ablative, 96
    applications of, 95
    carbon dioxide, 95, 96, 97
    categories of, 96
    CoolTouch, 137
    deep resurfacing, 97
    Erbium:YAG, 96, 97
    in spider vein treatments, 135
    infrared, 98
    Nlite, 137
    nonablative, 95, 98
    noninvasive, 54
    photorejuvenation, 96
    repigmenting, 100
    visible light, 98
Laser resurfacing, 63, 92, 93, 129, 130
Latino skin, 64
Lecithin, 38
LEDs, (see light-emitting diodes)